ESSENTIALS OF SURGICAL CRITICAL CARE

# CLINICAL CASES AND PRACTICAL SOLUTIONS

ESSENTIALS OF SURGICAL CRITICAL CARE

# CLINICAL CASES AND PRACTICAL SOLUTIONS

EDITED BY

**Jerome H. Abrams, M.D.**

Assistant Professor of Surgery and Associate Director of Critical Care, Department of Surgery, University of Minnesota; Staff Surgeon, Minneapolis VA Medical Center, Minneapolis, Minnesota

**Frank B. Cerra, M.D.**

Professor of Surgery, Department of Surgery, University of Minnesota; Director of Surgical Critical Care and Director of Nutritional Support Services, University of Minnesota Hospital and Clinic, Minneapolis, Minnesota, and St. Paul–Ramsey Medical Center, St. Paul, Minnesota

QMP

QUALITY MEDICAL PUBLISHING, INC

ST. LOUIS, MISSOURI 1993

Every effort has been made to ensure the accuracy of the drug dosages listed in this book; however, the health care professional is legally responsible for verifying the indications and dosage requirements with the manufacturers' package inserts and is thus advised.



Printed in the United States of America.

PUBLISHER Karen Berger
PROJECT MANAGER Carlotta Seely
PRODUCTION Shelley Zinselmeier
DESIGN Diane M. Beasley

Quality Medical Publishing, Inc.
11970 Borman Drive, Suite 222
St. Louis, Missouri 63146

LIBRARY OF CONGRESS CATALOGING-IN-PUBLICATION DATA

Essentials of surgical critical care—Clinical cases and practical solutions / edited by Jerome H. Abrams, Frank B. Cerra.
p. cm.
Includes bibliographical references.
ISBN 0-942219-32-5 (case book : pbk.)
1. Surgical intensive care—Case studies. 2. Critical care medicine—Case studies. 3. Therapeutics, Surgical—Case studies. I. Abrams, Jerome H., 1949- . II. Cerra, Frank B.
[DNLM: 1. Critical Illness—therapy—case studies. 2. Intensive Care—methods. 3. Surgery—case studies. WX 218 E782]
RD51.5.E772 1993
617'.919—dc20
DNLM/DLC
for Library of Congress 92-48762
CIP

GW/M/M

5 4 3 2 1

# CONTRIBUTORS

**Jerome H. Abrams,** M.D.
Assistant Professor of Surgery and
Associate Director of Critical Care,
Department of Surgery,
University of Minnesota;
Staff Surgeon,
Minneapolis VA Medical Center,
Minneapolis, Minnesota

**David H. Ahrenholz,** M.D.
Assistant Professor,
Department of Surgery,
University of Minnesota,
Minneapolis, Minnesota;
Associate Director, Burn Unit,
St. Paul–Ramsey Medical Center,
St. Paul, Minnesota

**Roderick A. Barke,** M.D.
Assistant Professor,
Department of Surgery,
University of Minnesota;
Director, Critical Care Units,
Minneapolis VA Medical Center,
Minneapolis, Minnesota

**Richard G. Barton,** M.D.
Assistant Professor of Surgery,
Department of Surgery,
University of Utah,
Salt Lake City, Utah

**Jon F. Berlauk,** M.D.
Assistant Professor of Anesthesiology,
Department of Anesthesiology, and
Assistant Director, SICU,
University of Minnesota,
Minneapolis, Minnesota

**Pamela K. Borchardt-Phelps,** Pharm.D.
Clinical Assistant Professor,
College of Pharmacy, and
Clinical Supervisor,
Department of Pharmaceutical Services,
University of Minnesota Hospital and Clinic,
Minneapolis, Minnesota

**Richard W. Carlson,** M.D., Ph.D.
Chairman and Professor of Medicine,
Department of Medicine,
University of Illinois College of Medicine,
Peoria, Illinois

**Frank B. Cerra,** M.D.
Professor of Surgery,
Department of Surgery,
University of Minnesota;
Director of Surgical Critical Care and
Director of Nutritional Support Services,
University of Minnesota Hospital and Clinic,
Minneapolis, Minnesota, and
St. Paul–Ramsey Medical Center,
St. Paul, Minnesota

**Mark D. Cipolle,** M.D., Ph.D.
Critical Care Fellow,
Department of Surgery,
University of Minnesota,
Minneapolis, Minnesota

**Vivian L. Clark,** M.D.
Clinical Instructor,
Department of Cardiology,
University of Michigan,
Ann Arbor, Michigan;
Senior Staff Cardiologist,
Henry Ford Hospital,
Detroit, Michigan

**Ricardo Correa-Rotter,** M.D.
Head, Department of Nephrology,
Instituto Nacional de la Nutrición/Salvador Zubiran,
Mexico City, Mexico

**Alan J. Cropp,** M.D.
Assistant Professor,
Northeastern Ohio Universities College of Medicine;
Assistant Director of Critical Care Medicine,
St. Elizabeth Hospital Medical Center,
Youngstown, Ohio

**Robert E. Cunnion,** M.D.
Senior Investigator and Chief,
Cardiovascular Section,
Department of Critical Care Medicine,
National Institutes of Health,
Bethesda, Maryland

**Elizabeth A. Davis,** M.D.
Assistant Professor,
Department of Physical Medicine and Rehabilitation,
University of Minnesota,
Minneapolis, Minnesota

**James P. Davison,** D.O.
Resident in Internal Medicine,
Department of Internal Medicine,
St. Elizabeth Hospital Medical Center,
Youngstown, Ohio

**R. Phillip Dellinger,** M.D., M.Sc.
Associate Professor and
Director of Critical Care,
Department of Medicine,
Baylor College of Medicine,
Houston, Texas

**Paul Druck,** M.D.
Clinical Instructor in Surgery,
Department of Surgery,
University of Minnesota,
Minneapolis, Minnesota

**David L. Dunn,** M.D., Ph.D.
Associate Professor of Surgery and
Head of Surgical Infectious Diseases,
Department of Surgery,
University of Minnesota,
Minneapolis, Minnesota

**David C. Evans,** M.D.
Chief Resident,
Department of Surgery,
McGill University,
Montreal, Quebec,
Canada

**Steven D. Eyer,** M.D.
Assistant Professor,
Department of Surgery,
University of Minnesota,
Minneapolis, Minnesota

**Martha A. Fehr,** M.D.
Staff Physician,
Department of Neurology,
University of Minnesota,
Minneapolis, Minnesota

**Barry W. Feig,** M.D.
Junior Faculty Associate,
Department of Surgery,
University of Texas M.D. Anderson Cancer Center,
Houston, Texas

**Ian J. Gilmour,** M.D.
Assistant Professor,
Department of Anesthesiology,
University of Minnesota,
Minneapolis, Minnesota

**Paul Gustafson,** R.N., C.R.T.T.
Cardiopulmonary Specialist,
Cardiopulmonary Services,
University of Minnesota Hospital and Clinic,
Minneapolis, Minnesota

**Guillermo Gutierrez,** M.D., Ph.D.
Professor,
Division of Pulmonary and Critical Care Medicine,
University of Texas Health Science Center Medical School,
Houston, Texas

**Marshall I. Hertz,** M.D.
Associate Professor,
Department of Internal Medicine,
University of Minnesota,
Minneapolis, Minnesota

**Steven M. Hollenberg**, M.D.
Senior Staff Fellow,
Department of Critical Care Medicine,
National Institutes of Health,
Bethesda, Maryland

**John W. Hoyt**, M.D.
Clinical Professor of Anesthesiology/Critical Care,
Department of Anesthesiology/Critical Care Medicine,
University of Pittsburgh,
Pittsburgh, Pennsylvania

**David S. Knopman**, M.D.
Associate Professor,
Department of Neurology,
University of Minnesota,
Minneapolis, Minnesota

**James A. Kruse**, M.D.
Associate Professor,
Division of Critical Care Medicine,
Wayne State University School of Medicine,
Detroit, Michigan

**Becky Jo Lekander**, R.N., M.S.N., C.C.R.N., C.S.
Clinical Nurse Specialist,
Department of Nursing Services,
University of Minnesota Hospital and Clinic,
Minneapolis, Minnesota

**Bruce C. Lohr**, Pharm.D.
Clinical Assistant Professor,
College of Pharmacy,
University of Minnesota;
Clinical Specialist,
Department of Pharmacy,
University of Minnesota Hospital and Clinic,
Minneapolis, Minnesota

**John E. Mazuski**, M.D.
Assistant Professor of Surgery,
Department of Surgery,
St. Louis University School of Medicine,
St. Louis, Missouri

**Jonathan L. Meakins**, M.D., D.Sc.
Professor and Chairman,
Department of Surgery,
McGill University,
Montreal, Quebec,
Canada

**Beth M. Nelson**, R.N., M.S.
Assistant Nurse Manager,
Department of Surgical Intensive Care,
University of Minnesota Hospital and Clinic,
Minneapolis, Minnesota

**Eric S. Nussbaum**, M.D.
Resident,
Department of Neurological Surgery,
University of Minnesota Hospital and Clinic,
Minneapolis, Minnesota

**Michael D. Pasquale**, M.D.
Critical Care Fellow,
Department of Surgery,
University of Minnesota,
Minneapolis, Minnesota

**Michael R. Pinsky**, M.D.
Professor and Director of Research,
Division of Critical Care Medicine,
Department of Anesthesiology and Critical Care Medicine,
University of Pittsburgh,
Pittsburgh, Pennsylvania

**Mark E. Rosenberg**, M.D.
Assistant Professor,
Division of Renal Diseases and Hypertension,
Department of Internal Medicine,
University of Minnesota,
Minneapolis, Minnesota

**Ori D. Rotstein**, M.D., F.R.C.S.(C), F.A.C.S.
Associate Professor,
Department of Surgery,
University of Toronto,
Toronto, Ontario,
Canada

**Leslie A. Sebring**, M.D., Ph.D.
Chief Resident,
Department of Neurological Surgery,
University of Minnesota Hospital and Clinic,
Minneapolis, Minnesota

**Richard L. Simmons**, M.D.
George V. Foster Professor of Surgery;
Associate Dean for Clinical Affairs,
School of Medicine;
Associate Vice-President for Clinical Affairs,
University of Pittsburgh Medical Center,
Pittsburgh, Pennsylvania

**Lynn D. Solem,** M.D.
Assistant Professor,
Department of Surgery,
University of Minnesota;
Director, Burn Unit,
St. Paul–Ramsey Medical Center,
St. Paul, Minnesota

**Oren K. Steinmetz,** M.D.
Fellow,
Department of Surgery,
McGill University,
Montreal, Quebec,
Canada

**Fernando Torres,** M.D.
Professor,
Department of Neurology,
University of Minnesota,
Minneapolis, Minnesota

**Gregory M. Vercellotti,** M.D.
Associate Professor,
Department of Internal Medicine,
University of Minnesota,
Minneapolis, Minnesota

**Kathleen V. Watson,** M.D.
Assistant Professor,
Department of Internal Medicine,
University of Minnesota,
Minneapolis, Minnesota

**Larry A. Woods,** D.O.
Assistant Professor of Internal Medicine,
Department of Internal Medicine,
Northeastern Ohio Universities College of Medicine;
Director, Critical Care Medicine,
St. Elizabeth Hospital Medical Center,
Youngstown, Ohio

**Carol H. Wysham,** M.D.
Department of Internal Medicine,
Rockwood Clinic,
Spokane, Washington

**Karl L. Yang,** M.D.
Assistant Professor,
Division of Pulmonary and Critical Care Medicine,
University of Texas Health Science Center,
Houston, Texas

# PREFACE

"Just the facts . . ." Not only fictitious detectives, but also practicing clinicians, long for the facts that will identify problems, clarify their solutions, and improve patient outcomes. Clinical problems present a recurrent theme. At best, the clinician can obtain only incomplete information, and, of the information available, a significant probability of error is associated with it. Nonetheless, when patients appear in the SICU, the tempo of their decompensation often is alarming. Although the clinician might very much lament the lack of complete and certain information about fulminant respiratory failure, for example, he or she cannot avoid the need for treating a patient in severe respiratory distress. Despite incompleteness of information, critical care practitioners use data, experience, and instinct to manage problems in the SICU. Data obtained from as clearly defined a group of patients as possible inform the treatment of similar patients. Experience allows the clinician to weigh the appropriateness of these data for application to individual patients. Although similar in many respects to the defined population, each patient presents unique demands. Finally, instinct helps chart new directions for diagnosis and treatment and opens new frontiers of research.

This collection of case studies is meant to stimulate your thinking. The cases, some relatively straightforward and others more complicated, are offered to help the reader apply the principles discussed in the companion volume to this book, *Essentials of Surgical Critical Care.** A rationale for managing the clinical problems is presented by each author. Note, *a* rationale, not *the* rationale, is offered. Clearly, different methods of approaching clinical problems exist. You may agree with the management presented in this book. If so, please keep track of patient outcomes to see if the diagnostic and treatment plans are appropriate for the kinds of patients you encounter. On the other hand, you may disagree with the management described here. If your disagreement sharpens your thoughts and improves your own approach, then this book will be even more useful. Please let us know about the improved methods that you discover. If your disagreement drives you to the laboratory to do research or leads you to design a clinical study to fill in the missing information, this book will have achieved its greatest purpose, and your discoveries will find an appreciative audience.

Presenting the cases and discussing them with your colleagues should increase their value. Reading this book aloud to groups of people should encourage different thoughts about the same problem. With many views expressed about the same problem, both the quantity and the quality of learning can only increase.

Ideally, this book will be used in conjunction with *Essentials of Surgical Critical Care.* Although each of the two books stands alone, each one can be used to its fullest potential along with the other volume. On the opening page of each chapter of this book, the main chapter reference in *Essentials of Surgical Critical Care* is indicated in a footnote; other chapters containing relevant information also are noted for the reader.

---

*Abrams JH, Cerra FB, eds. Essentials of Surgical Critical Care. St. Louis: Quality Medical Publishing, Inc., 1993.

A word about the format is helpful. The presentation of each case is shown in sans serif type. Discussion of the case information is shown in serif type. A list of the abbreviations used in the case presentations and discussions can be found at the end of this book.

This book represents an experiment in teaching the principles of critical care. We are indebted to the contributors for their imaginative and authoritative case studies. Having the benefit of their analyses of these interesting case presentations has broadened our own understanding of critical care.

We wish to thank Professor John S. Najarian for his continuing support of the surgical critical care program at the University of Minnesota. We also want to thank the staff of Quality Medical Publishing, Inc., for their expert help, enthusiastic support, and encouragement. Carlotta Seely of QMP perceived the structure of this work and transformed the endless collection of fragments into a coherent whole. Joan M. Johnson, of the Department of Surgery at the University of Minnesota, used her outstanding organizational and problem-solving skills to smooth the inevitably bumpy path from a hazy idea to a useful book. Without both of you, Carlotta and Joan, neither *Essentials of Surgical Critical Care* nor this book would exist. One of the great privileges of editing these volumes has been the chance to be a part of a team involved in the complicated effort of making a book succeed. To all the members of that team, we offer our sincere thanks.

**Jerome H. Abrams**
**Frank B. Cerra**

# CONTENTS

## PART ONE

## *ALTERED METABOLISM OF CRITICAL ILLNESS AND SHOCK*



## PART TWO

## *CARE OF THE CRITICALLY ILL PATIENT*

### SECTION 1

### Preoperative, Intraoperative, and Postoperative Evaluation



### SECTION 2

### Guidelines for Pharmacologic Problem-Solving

# PART THREE

# *PATHOPHYSIOLOGIC CONDITIONS*

## SECTION 1

### Central Nervous System



## SECTION 2

### Cardiovascular Function



## SECTION 3

### Pulmonary Function



## SECTION 4

### Renal Function



## SECTION 5

### Gastrointestinal and Hepatic Function



## SECTION 6

### Endocrine System

## PART FOUR
# *SYSTEMIC DYSFUNCTION*



## PART FIVE
# *COMMON SICU PROCEDURES*



## PART SIX
# *MEASUREMENT AND INTERPRETATION OF DATA*



## PART SEVEN
# *THE ART OF PRACTICE*

PART ONE

# *ALTERED METABOLISM OF CRITICAL ILLNESS AND SHOCK*

# CHAPTER 1

## *Restoration of Oxygen Transport*

Jerome H. Abrams

### CASE 1

A 19-year-old man was admitted to the emergency department following a motor vehicle accident. He was the driver of a motorcycle and sustained a collision with an automobile. On admission, bilateral pulmonary contusions and bilateral rib fractures were noted on the CXR films. Fluid in both the right chest and the left chest was seen. Ribs 2 to 5 were fractured on the right, and ribs 3 to 8 were fractured on the left. After it had been determined that the cervical spine was not injured, the patient was intubated. X-ray films of the pelvis and the extremities demonstrated a pelvic fracture and a left femur fracture. Bilateral chest tubes were placed, and approximately 350 ml of blood from the right side and 300 ml of blood from the left side was recovered. An intravenous pyelogram was obtained and demonstrated bilateral function and no obstruction. A cystourethrogram revealed no injury.

The patient was then taken to the operating room. Diagnostic peritoneal lavage was positive, and the patient underwent exploration. A liver laceration was noted. Examination of the liver revealed a single bleeding vessel that was ligated. The spleen was ruptured, and a splenectomy was performed. The transverse colon was lacerated. The lacerated section was resected, and an end-on colostomy and mucous fistula were constructed. The patient had a right perirenal hematoma, which, on observation, was not expanding. The pelvic fracture was stabilized with external fixators. A left femur fracture also was stabilized with an external fixator. No evidence of rectal injury was noted. Six hours postoperatively the patient's urine output was 15 ml/hr for 2 hours.

In a patient with multiple trauma, decreased urine output may be caused by several mechanisms. In a general way, oliguria may be a result of obstruction, renal causes, or prerenal causes. According to the patient's intravenous pyelogram, both kidneys were functioning and there was no evidence of obstruction. In addition, the cystogram demonstrated that the urinary bladder was also intact. Urinary electrolytes and creatinine will help to distinguish prerenal from renal causes. Fractional excretion of sodium then can be calculated. Prerenal mechanisms of oliguria include intravascular volume depletion as a consequence of hemorrhage, third-space losses, and cardiac insufficiency. A patient with blunt injury to the chest is at risk for cardiac contusion. CPKs with MB fractions should be obtained to assess the possibility of myocardial injury. In addition, such a patient should receive continuous ECG monitoring. A possible consequence of blunt chest injury is traumatic cardiac tamponade. The patient should be evaluated by physical

This chapter can be studied in conjunction with *Essentials of Surgical Critical Care,* edited by Jerome H. Abrams and Frank B. Cerra (St. Louis: Quality Medical Publishing, Inc., 1993), Chapters 1, *2,* 3, 4, and 5. Italicized number indicates the main chapter reference.

examination, with attention given to loudness and quality of the heart sounds, evidence of jugular venous distention, and pulsus paradoxicus, to determine the possibility of cardiac tamponade. If echocardiography is available, it may be of great assistance in establishing the presence or absence of wall motion abnormalities or pericardial fluid. The hemoglobin concentration should be measured, although acutely it may not reflect bleeding.

No physical evidence of cardiac tamponade was present on physical examination. The patient had no external signs of bleeding from the GI tract. In this patient the fractional excretion of sodium was $<1$, a finding consistent with prerenal causes. With the decreased fractional excretion of sodium, the potential for third-space losses, and the absence of cardiac reasons for oliguria, the patient was given intravascular fluid with a working diagnosis of intravascular volume depletion as a result of third-space losses. Lactated Ringer's solution (1.5 L) was administered without any demonstrable change in the patient's vital signs or urine output.

- *What is your approach at this time?*

Once again, the patient should be evaluated for clinical evidence of cardiac failure. If such evidence is not present, the possibility that he may continue to have intravascular volume depletion remains likely. Should additional intravenous fluids be administered? Are the available data satisfactory for a decision, or would additional information be helpful? Of greater significance, is the most important concern at this time the patient's volume status? With multiple trauma, this patient is at risk for developing multiple system organ failure. Along with source control, resuscitation by oxygen transport standards, followed by adequate metabolic support, is associated with decreased mortality. The patient already has had sources of injury controlled. To reduce mortality, the next mandate is to ensure adequate restoration of oxygen transport. With currently available technology, invasive hemodynamic monitoring is required to optimize oxygen transport. The idea of restoring oxygen transport does not mean that optimizing renal function has no clinical importance at this time. Rather, resuscitating patients by oxygen transport standards often simultaneously optimizes specific organ function. For the major indication of restoring oxygen transport, a pulmonary artery catheter is placed.

A pulmonary catheter was placed, and the following data were obtained:

| P | BP | UO | CO/CI | PCWP | $Do_2$ | $Dvo_2$ | $\dot{V}o_2$ | SVR | Hb | Lac |
|---|---|---|---|---|---|---|---|---|---|---|
| 140 | 80/55 | 15 | 4.2/2.5 | 4 | 523 | 5.8 | 144 | 1856 | 9.3 | 6.2 |

- *What information is needed to develop an adequate strategy for managing this patient?*

Since the pulmonary artery catheter is placed to assess the adequacy of resuscitation by oxygen transport standards, the following information is required: cardiac output, arterial oxygen saturation, venous oxygen saturation, arteriovenous oxygen content difference, pulmonary capillary wedge pressure, serum lactate concentration (or lactate/pyruvate ratio, if available), and hemoglobin concentration. With these data, one can calculate systemic vascular resistance, oxygen delivery, and oxygen consumption. In this patient the pulse is 140, and the blood pressure is 80/55. The cardiac index is 2.5, the pulmonary capillary wedge pressure is 4 mm Hg, the arteriovenous oxygen content difference is 5.8%, the hemoglobin is 9.3 g/dl, and the serum lactate is 4.2 mmol. With these data, the oxygen consumption is noted to be 149 ml/min/m$^2$ and the oxygen delivery is 523 ml/min. The systemic vascular resistance (SVR) is calculated to be 1900 dyne · sec · cm$^{-5}$.

- *Does the patient have flow-dependent oxygen consumption? Is lactate production flow-dependent?*

If the pyruvate is available, one can ask if the lactate/pyruvate ratio is $<20$. In this patient the lactate is 6.2 mmol. Clearly, the patient has not been resuscitated by oxygen transport standards. The lactate concentration is elevated. The arteriovenous oxygen content difference is wider than normal, a finding that suggests that the patient is extracting oxygen maximally. In addition, the oxygen consumption is below what one would expect for a patient with multiple injuries. The cardiac output is in the low normal range but is appropriate only for a patient who is nonstressed. The patient has the hallmarks of flow-dependent oxygen consumption. The goal should be to increase oxygen delivery and determine if oxygen consumption improves. First, adequacy of oxygen carriers (Hb) is assessed. Once adequate oxygen saturation has been ensured, cardiac output is optimized in order of preload, afterload, and contractility.

Since the patient had increased oxygen-carrying needs and was clearly at the low range of filling pressures, two units of packed red cells were transfused. The hemoglobin increased to 11.2 g/dl, and the pulmonary capillary wedge pressure increased to 12 mm Hg. The cardiac output increased to 14.6 L/min, and the cardiac index was 8.6 L/min/m$^2$. The oxygen delivery was then 2250 ml/min, and the oxygen consumption rose to 344 ml/min/m$^2$. The lactate fell to 1.6, and the blood pressure was 110/72. The patient's urine output increased to 60 ml/hr. The patient appeared to meet the requirements for resuscitation by oxygen transport standards. The arteriovenous oxygen content difference was in the target range. The pulmonary capillary wedge pressure was in the target range, and the lactate was normalized. The oxygen consumption was well above that expected for a patient with polytrauma.

| P | BP | UO | CO/CI | PCWP | $Do_2$ | $Dvo_2$ | $\dot{V}o_2$ | SVR | Hb | Lac |
|---|---|---|---|---|---|---|---|---|---|---|
| 90 | 110/72 | 50 | 14.6/8.6 | 12 | 2250 | 4 | 344 | 810 | 11.8 | 1.6 |

The patient continued to do well until postoperative day 5. At that time the patient's pulse was 125, and his blood pressure was 85/10. The urine output decreased to 0.5 ml/kg/hr. The patient had a temperature of 102.4° F. His skin was warm and capillary refill was normal. He complained of increasing abdominal tenderness. The serum amylase and lipase concentrations both were markedly elevated. A CT scan of the abdomen revealed an edematous pancreas, and a diagnosis of acute pancreatitis was made.

The following information was obtained:

| P | BP | UO | CO/CI | PCWP | $Do_2$ | $Dvo_2$ | $\dot{V}o_2$ | SVR | Hb | Lac |
|---|---|---|---|---|---|---|---|---|---|---|
| 125 | 85/60 | 35 | 8.8/5.2 | 8 | 1468 | 2.9 | 150 | 777 | 10.2 | 4.6 |

The patient is not resuscitated by oxygen transport standards, as he was earlier. The findings of a narrowed arteriovenous oxygen content difference and decreased SVR are consistent with the diagnosis of acute pancreatitis. Again, the mandate is to increase oxygen delivery and determine whether oxygen consumption increases. The patient does not meet the target for pulmonary capillary wedge pressure, and the hemoglobin is 10.2 g/dl. Accordingly, since his need for increased oxygen carrying capacity remains, preload, in the form of packed RBCs, is administered. The following data are obtained:

| P | BP | UO | CO/CI | PCWP | $Do_2$ | $Dvo_2$ | $\dot{V}o_2$ | SVR | Hb | Lac |
|---|---|---|---|---|---|---|---|---|---|---|
| 110 | 94/65 | 40 | 11.3/6.6 | 14 | 1755 | 2.6 | 172 | 682 | 11.9 | 4.1 |

The hemoglobin rises to 11.5 g/dl, the cardiac output increases to 11.3 L/min, with a cardiac index of 6.6 $L \cdot min^{-1} \cdot m^{-2}$. The pulmonary catheter wedge pressure is 14 mm Hg, and oxygen delivery increases to 1755 ml/min. The arteriovenous oxygen content remains the same: 2.6 vol%. The oxygen consumption is 172 ml · $min^{-1}$ · $m^{-2}$, and the SVR is 682. Lactate is 4.1 mmol. The cardiac index and oxygen consumption are increased but are not as high as on the first postoperative night. The oxygen consumption is nearly 180 ml · $min^{-1}$· $m^{-2}$, a value consistent with the highest level of metabolic stress. The elevated lactate concentration suggests that in this patient, who has multiple trauma and acute pancreatitis, increased oxygen delivery and consumption are necessary. Since the hemoglobin concentration is adequate and preload has been restored, the next variable to consider is afterload. The SVR of 682 is well below the target range. Since the patient appears to need more oxygen delivery, further reduction of SVR with vasodilators is unlikely to be well tolerated or to cause a significant increase in oxygen delivery. Inotropic support should be considered.

Accordingly, dobutamine was added to the patient's regimen. The following information was obtained:

| P | BP | UO | CO/CI | PCWP | $Do_2$ | $Dvo_2$ | $\dot{V}o_2$ | SVR | Hb | Lac |
|---|---|---|---|---|---|---|---|---|---|---|
| 120 | 115/64 | 45 | 13.6/8 | 12 | 2042 | 2.5 | 201 | 630 | 11.5 | 1.4 |

With this intervention, cardiac output increases to 13.6 and the cardiac index is 8. The pulmonary capillary wedge pressure is 12 mm Hg, and the oxygen delivery is 2042 ml/min. The arterio-venous oxygen delivery difference is nearly unchanged, at 2.5%. The hemoglobin is 11.5. The lactate is normal at 1.4 mmol. The calculated variable, oxygen consumption index at 201 ml · $min^{-1}$· $m^{-2}$, is appropriate for the patient's clinical state. The SVR is virtually unchanged at 630. An increase in $Do_2$ of 16% was associated with an increase in $\dot{V}o_2$ of 17%. Augmenting oxygen transport in this manner was associated with reducing the serum lactate concentration to normal. By the criteria of oxygen transport, the patient appears to be adequately resuscitated.

## CASE 2

A 39-year-old woman was admitted for elective cholecystectomy. Laparotomy and cholecystectomy were performed for cholelithiasis. The procedures were uncomplicated. The patient's estimated blood loss was negligible, and the bile obtained from the gallbladder was sent for Gram's stain and culture. The patient had no significant medical history and was taking no medications preoperatively. She was extubated routinely in the postanesthesia recovery unit. During the first postoperative night, she received family visitors, who noted that she was progressing well.

You were telephoned at 3:00 AM of the first postoperative night because the patient was then disoriented. You immediately went to see the patient. She was disoriented for place and time but orientated for person. Her temperature was 101.2° F, blood pressure was 120/80, heart rate was 110, and respiratory rate was 28. The lungs were clear on percussion and auscultation, the cardiac examination was normal, and the abdominal examination revealed only incisional tenderness. The skin disclosed no abnormalities, with the exception of the new incision. The new incision was examined, and the wound was noted as unremarkable. A detailed neurologic examination revealed no additional focal neurologic deficit.

- *What is your approach at this point?*

The appearance of disorientation and tachypnea in this patient is worrisome. Disorientation with tachypnea and acute respiratory alkalosis are the earliest signs of Gram-negative sepsis.

Although a Gram's stain and culture of the bile were obtained at the time of the operative procedure, currently no information about whether bacteria were present is on hand. This patient should be treated for Gram-negative sepsis while the evaluation continues. Administration of antibiotics that are appropriate for Gram-negative pathogens of the biliary tree should be instituted immediately. For this patient a third-generation cephalosporin and metronidazole were selected.

With the working diagnosis of Gram-negative sepsis, intravenous hydration was begun with lactated Ringer's solution. Laboratory results showed that the Gram's stain revealed many Gram-negative rods in the bile. Despite administration of 2 L of lactated Ringer's solution over approximately 45 minutes, the patient's blood pressure fell from 120/80 to 90/60. In addition, her heart rate increased from 110 to 140. The rhythm was regular. A repeat oral temperature was 102.7° F. The respiratory rate remained elevated at 32. An arterial blood gas study confirmed the suspicion that respiratory alkalosis was present. The pH was 7.52, the $Paco_2$ was 28, and $Pao_2$ was 110 while the patient was breathing 2 L/min oxygen via nasal cannula. Blood samples were sent for CBC, electrolytes, and coagulation studies. Cultures of blood and urine were obtained.

- *What is your approach at this point?*

These findings are all consistent with Gram-negative septic shock. Your main concern at this point should be the management of septic shock. Fluid replacement with colloid should be started immediately. Although controversy exists about the relative advantages of crystalloid vs. colloid, nearly all practitioners agree that physiologic endpoints should guide volume replacement therapy. You decide to transfer the patient to an SICU at this time with a working diagnosis of Gram-negative septic shock. The indication for transporting the patient to the SICU is resuscitation from shock according to the criteria for restoration of oxygen transport. It is clear that this patient requires resuscitation. In this case resuscitation means not simply maintenance of blood pressure and reduction of the pulse, but resuscitation by the standards of oxygen transport. These standards of adequate resuscitation include absence of flow-dependent oxygen consumption and absence of flow-dependent lactate production, a normalization of the lactate/pyruvate ratio. With our current abilities, invasive hemodynamic monitoring is necessary to obtain the information necessary for assessing oxygen transport. In this situation, blood pressure, pulse, urine output, capillary refill, and mental status are neither sensitive nor specific for assessing restoration of oxygen transport.

With colloid infusion ongoing, the patient was transferred to the SICU. A pulmonary artery catheter and an arterial line were placed. By this time, several laboratory test results were available. The hemoglobin was 11.5, electrolytes were normal, and coagulation studies also were normal. The following variables were measured:

| P | BP | UO | CO/CI | PCWP | $Do_2$ | $Dvo_2$ | $\dot{V}o_2$ | SVR | Hb | Lac |
|---|---|---|---|---|---|---|---|---|---|---|
| 110 | 85/52 | 40 | 5.5/3.2 | 4 | 826 | 2.9 | 93 | 766 | 11.5 | 6.2 |

The hemodynamic data obtained suggest that this patient requires additional preload. Although the patient's pulmonary capillary wedge pressure is normal, she demonstrates inadequate oxygen transport. The derived $\dot{V}o_2$ is low for her clinical situation, and the lactate concentration is 6.5 mmol. The arteriovenous content difference is below normal. This finding is consistent with sepsis and is characteristic of a global oxygen extraction deficit. The SVR also is consistent with septic shock.

With an elevated serum lactate concentration ratio and the question of whether flow-dependent oxygen consumption is present, the mandate is to increase oxygen delivery and assess the changes. The most efficient intervention is restoring the oxygen carrying capacity by maintaining adequate hemoglobin concentration. This patient's hemoglobin concentration is probably adequate. Although her pulse is slightly elevated, she demonstrates no evidence of cardiac ischemia. At this time the risks of transfusion outweigh the potential benefits. Increasing cardiac output at this point is the next appropriate step for increasing oxygen delivery. Cardiac output should be optimized in terms of preload, afterload, and, finally, contractility. The patient's capillary wedge pressure is currently 6 mm Hg. With acute sepsis, myocardial dysfunction may be present. Increasing preload may augment cardiac output.

Additional colloid was infused until the wedge pressure reached 14 mm Hg. At this point, another hemodynamic profile was obtained.

| P | BP | UO | CO/CI | PCWP | $Do_2$ | $Dvo_2$ | $\dot{V}o_2$ | SVR | Hb | Lac |
|---|---|---|---|---|---|---|---|---|---|---|
| 110 | 90/55 | 45 | 7.2/4.2 | 14 | 1071 | 2.8 | 119 | 655 | 11.4 | 4.1 |

- *What interventions will you make at this point?*

The increase in preload produces a concomitant increase in oxygen delivery. With the increased oxygen delivery, the patient's oxygen consumption also increases. The lactate concentration, nonetheless, remains abnormally high. This patient does not yet meet the current criteria for resuscitation by oxygen transport standards. She has hyperlacticacidemia and flow-dependent oxygen consumption. The mandate remains to increase oxygen delivery and determine the changes in the patient's oxygen transport and consumption. Preload now meets the target values. Next afterload is addressed. Afterload, as measured by SVR, is well below the usual clinical target. This finding is consistent with the diagnosis of Gram-negative sepsis. Most likely, further vasodilation would not be effective. In addition, hypotension and inadequate splanchnic organ perfusion from further vasodilation might occur. At this point increased contractility should be effected with an inotropic agent.

Dobutamine infusion was started. The infusion was rapidly increased to the level of 10 μg/kg/min. Once this dose had been achieved, a new hemodynamic profile was obtained, with the following results:

| P | BP | UO | CO/CI | PCWP | $Do_2$ | $Dvo_2$ | $\dot{V}o_2$ | SVR | Hb | Lac |
|---|---|---|---|---|---|---|---|---|---|---|
| 100 | 95/55 | 45 | 11.4/6.7 | 14 | 1747 | 2.8 | 108 | 436 | 11.5 | 1.8 |

With the increase in contractility, both oxygen delivery and oxygen consumption increase. With increased oxygen delivery, a concomitant decrease in serum lactate has been obtained. The patient's arteriovenous oxygen content difference did not change very much during the resuscitation effort. The global oxygen extraction deficit has been persistent throughout this period of resuscitation. The approach to this patient is comparable to that for the patient with multiple trauma in Case 1. In the present case, afterload reduction was not indicated. Although the algorithm remains essentially the same, the individual therapeutic decisions vary with the patient's underlying diagnosis and response to therapy.

By postoperative day 4, the patient had a stable blood pressure, pulse, and respiratory rate while on mechanical ventilation. She maintained a pH of 7.43, a $Paco_2$ of 36 mm Hg, and a $Pao_2$ of 110 mm Hg. The hemoglobin remained at 11.8 g/dl. Nonetheless, lactate concentration had increased to 2.8 mmol. At this time another hemodynamic profile was obtained:

| P | BP | UO | CO/CI | PCWP | $Do_2$ | $Dvo_2$ | $\dot{V}o_2$ | SVR | Hb | Lac |
|---|---|---|---|---|---|---|---|---|---|---|
| 100 | 98/55 | 45 | 8.7/5.1 | 14 | 1368 | 2.8 | 143 | 584 | 11.8 | 2.8 |

The oxygen consumption is less than that of the first postoperative night. The lactate concentration, however, is somewhat above the limits of normal. Because of the worry that the patient is now only partly resuscitated and may be in a flow-dependent oxygen consumption state, the goal is to improve oxygen delivery and assess the effects on oxygen consumption. Dobutamine infusion therapy is reinstituted to further augment oxygen delivery. Inotropic support is provided because the preload has been maintained and the patient is unlikely to tolerate further afterload reduction. Her SVR is well below the usual clinical target.

Dobutamine infusion was again instituted. The infusion rate was increased to 10 mg/kg/min. Another hemodynamic profile was obtained, with these data shown:

| P | BP | UO | CO/CI | PCWP | $Do_2$ | $Dvo_2$ | $\dot{V}o_2$ | SVR | Hb | Lac |
|---|---|---|---|---|---|---|---|---|---|---|
| 110 | 102/58 | 45 | 12.2/7.2 | 13 | 1869 | 2.3 | 165 | 453 | 11.5 | 2.7 |

With oxygen delivery increasing by nearly 50%, the oxygen consumption increases marginally. Nonetheless, the serum lactate concentration remains unchanged. An alternate possibility is that the patient's metabolism is best described by aerobic glycolysis. Current thinking about this condition is that entry of pyruvate into tricarboxcylic acid cycle is reduced because pyruvate dehydrogenase (PDH) is down-regulated. ATP production remains normal because other sources of carbon are used for energy production. Clinically, a test of this hypothesis is the measurement of the serum lactate/pyruvate ratio. Accordingly, a serum sample is obtained for determination of the lactate/pyruvate ratio.

The serum lactate/pyruvate ratio information was returned, and the value was noted as 16.7.

These findings are consistent with sepsis and aerobic glycolysis. Increased oxygen delivery did not produce a large increase in oxygen consumption, as measured by the indirect Fick method. In particular, increased oxygen delivery did not affect the serum lactate concentration. Nonetheless, the serum lactate/pyruvate ratio is within normal limits. These findings suggest that little additional benefit can be obtained from increasing oxygen delivery further. At this point, the patient has been resuscitated as far as possible by oxygen transport standards. This patient's course is consistent with that of a subset of patients who have persistent mild hyperlacticacidemia despite increased oxygen delivery. In such patients the lactate/pyruvate ratio is helpful in determining whether further resuscitation by oxygen transport standards is necessary.

# CHAPTER 2

# *Nutritional and Metabolic Support*

Frank B. Cerra

## CASE 1

A 38-year-old man was admitted to the SICU with severe pancreatitis that was complicated by adult respiratory distress syndrome. He required mechanical ventilation. An admission evaluation revealed the following:

| | | |
|---|---|---|
| Temperature: 102° F | Weight: 70 kg | Bilirubin: 3.2 mg/dl |
| $\dot{V}O_2$: 190 ml · min$^{-1}$ · m$^{-2}$ | Albumin: 2.6 g/dl | BUN: 20 mg/dl |
| Glucose: 130 mg/dl | Transferrin: 180 mg/dl | Creatinine: 0.9 mg/dl |
| R/Q: 0.83 | Nitrogen balance: −17 g/day | TUN: 15 g/day |

Because of a lack of enteral access past the pylorus and the presence of gastric atony, parenteral nutrition was chosen for nutritional support. On clinical examination, the body composition appeared to be normal. The low levels of albumin and transferrin reflected sequestration and a relative decrease in hepatic production. The high $\dot{V}O_2$ and marked negative nitrogen balance reflected a high degree of metabolic stress. The combination of increased energy expenditure, the probability of a long SICU stay with persistent hypermetabolism, the high risk of single and generalized nutrient deficiencies, and rapid catabolism of the lean body mass requires nutritional support based on the metabolic principles of hypermetabolic, mediated clinical states to prevent acquired starvation malnutrition from adding comorbidity or comortality.

| Category of Stress | Calories (kcal/day) | Carbohydrate (g/day) | Fat as Long-Chain Triglyceride (g/day) | Amino Acids as BcAA-Enriched Solution (g/day) |
|---|---|---|---|---|
| Maximum | 2100 | 350 | 70 | 105 |

Since the patient had adequate renal function, no volume restriction was necessary. Therefore 2000 ml was chosen as TPN volume exclusive of fat. This volume will fit into one bag, which offers a major cost savings. The intravenous fat was piggybacked at the IV port closest to the central line entrance site. The formula ordered was 17.5% glucose in 5.1% branched-chain amino acid (BcAA)–enriched solution administered at 50 ml/hr for 6 hours, then 75 ml/hr for 8 hours, and then 80 ml/hr. To this formula was added 0.5% normal saline solution, 10 mg/L zinc, 10 mEq/L magnesium, trace element solution, and Multiple Vitamin Insert for adults; 250 ml of 20% intravenous fat was ordered at 10 ml/hr. This formula provided 17 g of protein nitrogen, resulting in a nonprotein calorie-to-nitrogen ratio of 104/1.

---

This chapter can be studied in conjunction with *Essentials of Surgical Critical Care,* edited by Jerome H. Abrams and Frank B. Cerra (St. Louis: Quality Medical Publishing, Inc., 1993), Chapters 1, 2, *3,* and 4. Italicized number indicates the main chapter reference.

Five days later, a 24-hour urine sample was collected, and blood chemistry tests were performed. The results were:

| | | |
|---|---|---|
| Temperature: 101.6° F | Weight: 74 kg | Bilirubin: 3.4 mg/dl |
| $\dot{V}O_2$: 180 ml · min$^{-1}$ · m$^{-2}$ | Albumin: 2.4 g/dl | BUN: 45 mg/dl |
| Glucose: 160 mg/dl | Transferrin: 160 mg/dl | Creatinine: 1.2 mg/dl |
| R/Q: 0.86 | Nitrogen balance: −7 g/day | TUN: 22 g/day |

Continued hypermetabolism was present. The effects of the TPN are evident in the level of blood glucose, R/Q, BUN, and TUN. The blood glucose concentration was sufficient without treatment. The nitrogen balance was calculated as follows:

*Nitrogen in:* 102 g amino acid/6 g nitrogen/g of amino acid formula yields 17 g nitrogen in
*Nitrogen out:* TUN of 22 g + 2 g skin and insensible and nasogastric tube losses yields 24 g nitrogen out
*Nitrogen balance:* Nitrogen in − nitrogen out = 17 − 24 = −7 g/day

To improve the negative nitrogen balance, the amino acid portion of the formula was adjusted to 7.5%. The remainder of the formula was left the same.

| Category of Stress | Calories (kcal/day) | Carbohydrate (g/day) | Fat as Long-Chain Triglyceride (g/day) | Amino Acids as BcAA-Enriched Solution (g/day) |
|---|---|---|---|---|
| Maximum | 2100 | 350 | 70 | 105 |
| Original formula | 2168 | 340 | 50 | 102 |
| Revised formula | 2360 | 340 | 50 | 150 |

The degree of hypermetabolism was reflected in the continued negative nitrogen balance and the persistence of a low level of plasma transferrin. The nitrogen intake was increased to offset the negative nitrogen balance. The new formula provided 25 g of nitrogen with a nonprotein calorie-to-nitrogen ratio of 70/1. The blood chemistry tests were repeated 5 days later.

| | | |
|---|---|---|
| Temperature: 101° F | Weight: 74 kg | Bilirubin: 3.8 mg/dl |
| $\dot{V}O_2$: 175 ml · min$^{-1}$ · m$^{-2}$ | Albumin: 2.4 g/dl | BUN: 65 mg/dl |
| Glucose: 180 mg/dl | Transferrin: 150 mg/dl | Creatinine: 1.4 mg/dl |
| R/Q: 0.84 | Nitrogen balance: −2 g/day | TUN: 25 g/day |

The formula corrections improved the nitrogen retention. The patient's condition and the trend in the blood chemistry results indicated the continued presence of, and probable worsening of, the inflammatory process. A CT scan demonstrated the presence of a pancreatic abscess. The patient was taken to surgery, and a pancreatic abscess was drained. A jejunal feeding tube was placed at that time and jejunal tube feedings were begun.

## CASE 2

A 24-year-old man who was the passenger in a motor vehicle accident sustained these injuries: midshaft left femur fracture, severe pancreaticoduodenal injury, and large left pulmonary contusion. The patient arrived at the emergency department in shock. Following resuscitation he was taken to the operating room. The pancreaticoduodenal injury was managed by a duodenal exclusion procedure, and a feeding jejunostomy was placed. The fractured femur was then repaired, and the patient was taken to the SICU and maintained on mechanical ventilation. Hemodynamic stability was achieved within several hours of entering the SICU. Enteral feedings were then begun. At this point, an evaluation showed the following:

| | | |
|---|---|---|
| Temperature: 100° F | Weight: 70 kg | Bilirubin: 1.5 mg/dl |
| $\dot{V}O_2$: 150 ml · min$^{-1}$ · m$^{-2}$ | Albumin: 2.8 g/dl | BUN: 10 mg/dl |
| Glucose: 130 mg/dl | Transferrin: 185 mg/dl | Creatinine: 0.9 mg/dl |
| Lactate: 1.9 mg/dl | Nitrogen balance: −14 g/day | TUN: 14 g/day estimated from 6 hr urine collection |

The feeding tube permits the immediate initiation of postoperative enteral feedings. Even though the enteral route has been observed to be safe and as nutritionally efficacious as the parenteral route, no definitive evidence that this route of administration is associated with better patient outcome has been demonstrated. However, small clinical trials, studies in experimental settings, and the consensus of most practitioners support the enteral route as more efficacious for patient outcome. The enteral feeding was delayed until hemodynamic stability and adequate resuscitation were achieved. Experimental evidence indicates that feeding during the shock state may be associated with adverse outcome.

The feedings were initiated full strength at 25 ml/hr for 6 hours, followed by 50 ml/hr for 6 hours, then 60 ml/hr for 6 hours. The maintenance rate was 70 ml/hr. The feedings were well tolerated.

Note that enteral products are manufactured such that a predetermined minimum volume contains the full complement of nutrients considered appropriate. Formulation is based on the patient group to be treated. In addition, most enteral products are complete: they contain not only the nutrients, but all the necessary known vitamins, trace elements, and minerals. Thus, to provide complete nutrition, the minimum volume must be administered. If only 60% is administered, semistarvation and nutrient deficiencies will develop.

The principles of nutrition in this setting apply for the hypermetabolic-mediated clinical state, independent of route of administration. Again, a low nonprotein calorie-to-nitrogen ratio (100/1) is associated with improved nitrogen retention and support of hepatocellular protein synthesis. The BcAA-enriched formulas also are associated with improved nitrogen retention. Formulas in which the major source of calories is glucose are associated with excess carbon dioxide production and many other problems. A number of formulas also contain fat calories in excess of 25% of total calories. Formulas with less than 25% long-chain fatty acids are probably more appropriate. Formulas enriched with glutamine have not demonstrated improved efficacy. In addition, most enteral formulas contain adequate amounts of glutamine.

Enteral formulas offer several advantages. Arginine, ribonucleic acids, and n-3 polyunsaturated fatty acids can be given by the enteral route. Medium-chain fatty acids, which may become available soon, also can be given enterally.

In the case under discussion, several risk factors indicated a high likelihood of a prolonged SICU stay. The response to such major injury can be immune suppression and an increased incidence of nosocomial infections. For these reasons, the enteral formula chosen was one enriched with arginine, n-3 fatty acids, and ribonucleic acids. This formula provides 1.1 kcal/ml, 65 g protein/L as lactalbumin, and comprises 24% fatty acids. Half is medium-chain fatty acid; half is long-chain fatty acid. Of long-chain fatty acid, approximately half is n-3 fatty acid.

Five days later, a 24-hour urine sample was collected, and blood chemistry tests were done again.

| | | |
|---|---|---|
| Temperature: 102.5° F | Weight: 74 kg | Bilirubin: 4.2 mg/dl |
| $\dot{V}O_2$: 175 ml · min$^{-1}$ · m$^{-2}$ | Albumin: 2.4 g/dl | BUN: 65 mg/dl |
| Glucose: 180 mg/dl | Transferrin: 150 mg/dl | Creatinine: 1.2 mg/dl |
| UUN: 16 g/dl | Nitrogen balance: −3.3 g/day | TUN: 23 g/day |

Determination of nitrogen balance is useful in enteral nutrition. This patient illustrates the discrepancy that can develop between UUN and TUN. The UUN usually underestimates the urine nitrogen excretion. Stool collections performed during enteral nutrition show that over 95% of the nitrogen administered is absorbed. This absorption cannot be predicted from the stool volume. Most diarrhea in SICU patients is secretory in origin, and the enteral feeds are well absorbed even in its presence. To adjust the nitrogen lost from stool losses in the nitrogen balance calculation, an additional 2 g is added, bringing the total to 4 g added to the TUN.

The formula rate was increased to a rate of 80 ml/hr and maintained at that rate throughout the SICU course.

## CASE 3

A 65-year-old man was admitted to the SICU with a ruptured aortic aneurysm, hypotension, and oliguria. He was taken to the operating room, his infrarenal aortic aneurysm was repaired, and he was returned to the SICU. The patient was extubated; his urine output was 125 ml/hr, and he was clinically well perfused. The results of the tests were:

| | | |
|---|---|---|
| Temperature: 100° F | Weight: 80 kg | Bilirubin: 1.5 mg/dl |
| $\dot{V}O_2$: 130 ml · min$^{-1}$ · m$^{-2}$ | Albumin: 2.8 g/dl | BUN: 10 mg/dl |
| Glucose: 130 mg/dl | Transferrin: 185 mg/dl | Creatinine: 1.8 mg/dl |
| Lactate: 3.1 mg/dl | Nitrogen balance: −12 g/day | TUN: 12 g/day (estimated from 6 hr urine collection) |

No metabolic support was instituted because the likelihood that the patient would eat in a few days was thought to be high. The next day, the test results were:

| | | |
|---|---|---|
| Temperature: 101° F | Weight: 83 kg | Bilirubin: 3.1 mg/dl |
| $\dot{V}O_2$: 200 ml · min$^{-1}$ · m$^{-2}$ | Albumin: 2.6 g/dl | BUN: 15 mg/dl |
| Glucose: 160 mg/dl | Transferrin: 145 mg/dl | Creatinine: 2.2 mg/dl |
| Lactate: 2.9 mg/dl | | |

This patient's treatment included increased oxygen delivery, but no increase in $\dot{V}O_2$ was demonstrated. The clinical picture that developed was consistent with acute lung injury, so the patient was intubated and placed on mechanical ventilation. After the patient's condition was stabilized, a feeding tube was passed into the duodenum with bedside fluoroscopy, and tube feedings were begun. In 36 hours, feedings were administered at full strength and full volume. A formula enriched with arginine, n-3 fatty acids, and ribonucleic acid was used and administered at a rate of 90 ml/hr. Four days later, the monitoring profile was repeated.

| | | |
|---|---|---|
| Temperature: 102° F | Weight: 85 kg | Bilirubin: 5.7 mg/dl |
| $\dot{V}O_2$: 225 ml · min$^{-1}$ · m$^{-2}$ | Albumin: 2.6 g/dl | BUN: 85 mg/dl |
| Glucose: 190 mg/dl | Transferrin: 145 mg/dl | Creatinine: 2.8 mg/dl |
| Lactate: 2.8 mg/dl | Nitrogen balance: +2.7 g/day | TUN: 14 g/day |

The patient developed systemic inflammatory response with multiple organ dysfunction. The positive nitrogen balance reflected the progressive reduction in glomerular filtration (nonsteady state) and the accumulation of urea nitrogen in the total body water. The patient also remained in a highly catabolic state, reflected in the magnitude of rise in the BUN. At this point, no indication to change the enteral formulation was present. Blood chemistry tests were repeated 5 days later.

| | | |
|---|---|---|
| Temperature: 102° F | Weight: 89 kg | Bilirubin: 6.4 mg/dl |
| $\dot{V}O_2$: 119 ml · min$^{-1}$ · m$^{-2}$ | Albumin: 2.6 g/dl | BUN: 217 mg/dl |
| Glucose: 190 mg/dl | Transferrin: 145 mg/dl | Creatinine: 4.2 mg/dl |
| Lactate: 2.5 mg/dl | Phosphorus: 6.5 mEq/L | Potassium: 5.9 mEq/L |
| Arterial pH: 7.3 | | |

The organ dysfunction has progressed. Continuous arteriovenous hemifiltration with dialysis was instituted, and the enteral feedings were continued. Over the next 7 days, the patient progressively improved. He survived and was discharged to home.

PART TWO

# *CARE OF THE CRITICALLY ILL PATIENT*

# SECTION 1 *Preoperative, Intraoperative, and Postoperative Evaluation*

## CHAPTER 3

# *Initial Approach to the Injured Patient*

Richard G. Barton

### CASE 1

A 25-year-old man was transported by helicopter to the emergency department after the automobile he was driving collided with an oncoming semitrailer. The combined speed of the two vehicles was reported to be in excess of 100 mph. The victim was apparently unconscious initially, but he was conscious, with a Glasgow Coma Scale score of 15, when paramedic personnel arrived on the scene. It took 50 minutes to extract the victim from the crushed passenger compartment of his car, and he was placed in a hard cervical collar and immobilized on a backboard as soon as it was feasible. Initial vital signs included a BP of 60 palpable, an HR of 135, and an RR of 24. The patient was noted to have obvious deformities of the left forearm and left thigh consistent with fractures of those extremities. A right antecubital IV line was placed, and 2 L of lactated Ringer's solution was administered en route to the hospital.

On arrival in the emergency department, the patient was awake and alert, complaining of pain in the neck, chest, upper abdomen, hips, and left forearm and thigh. Vital signs on arrival (after administration of 2 L of crystalloid) were BP 80/50, HR 120, and RR 24. A brief initial examination revealed symmetrical breath sounds, contusions and abrasions over the anterior chest and upper abdomen, abdominal tenderness and voluntary guarding but no obvious distention, severe pain and instability on rocking of the hips and pelvis, and open fractures of the left ulna and radius and left femur. Distal pulses were thready or absent in all extremities.

- *How would you proceed at this point?*

In a patient with multiple injuries, the first steps are always to maintain the airway, support or assist breathing, and support or maintain the circulation, while protecting the patient against permanent neurologic injury. This patient was breathing, although somewhat rapidly, and in no serious respiratory distress. Face-mask oxygen would be adequate for the present. The

This chapter can be studied in conjunction with *Essentials of Surgical Critical Care,* edited by Jerome H. Abrams and Frank B. Cerra (St. Louis: Quality Medical Publishing, Inc., 1993), Chapter 5.

patient's most life-threatening problem was hypotension and apparent circulatory shock. Only one IV line was in place; a second one should be placed and aggressive fluid resuscitation should be continued without delay.

Because the patient's uncatheterized left upper extremity appeared to be fractured, a right saphenous vein cutdown was performed, a 12-gauge angiocatheter was placed, and an additional 2 L of warmed crystalloid was rapidly infused. Blood samples were drawn and sent for type and crossmatch and for laboratory tests. With the infusion of 2 L of crystalloid, the patient's BP rose to 110/60, and his HR fell to 105. Peripheral pulses were then present in all extremities.

With his circulation restored, the patient was undressed, and a more thorough history and physical examination were performed. He denied drug allergies and underlying medical problems. The chest and abdominal examinations were as noted previously. Extensive hematoma was noted in the left thigh and forearm. Both extremities were intact from a neurovascular standpoint, although the left lower extremity appeared foreshortened. On rectal examination, the prostate was difficult to palpate and seemed to be surrounded by hematoma. Stool was guaiac negative.

Chest and lateral cervical spine x-ray films were obtained and sent to be developed. A nasogastric tube was placed. An anteroposterior x-ray film of the pelvis was also obtained.

- *What should you do while waiting for the x-ray films to be developed?*

The abnormal rectal examination — specifically, the hematoma surrounding the prostate gland — suggested urethral injury, presumed to be secondary to the suspected pelvic fracture. Blood in the stool might suggest a rectal tear or perforation, also secondary to the suspected pelvic fracture. A Foley catheter should not be placed until a retrograde urethrogram confirms an intact urethra.

A fracture of the forearm should be immobilized with an appropriate splint. A commercially available pneumatic splint can be used until time permits the placement of a better one. When the fracture is open (compound), the patient will need to go to the operating room for irrigation, debridement, and probable external fixation.

An open fracture of the femur also requires operative debridement and fixation but can be stabilized in a Hare traction splint to control bleeding and minimize tissue injury until operative stabilization can be performed.

The lateral cervical spine x-ray film was returned to the trauma suite, and the spine appeared to be intact to C-6.

The anteroposterior CXR film is shown in Fig. 3-1.

- *What is your evaluation at this time?*

The lateral cervical spine film is inadequate, and a "swimmer's view" should be obtained, if possible, before manipulation of the neck is considered (e.g., intubation for anesthesia). The patient also requires completion of the C-spine series, including anteroposterior and odontoid views, which can be done when conditions permit. In addition, because of the patient's initial complaints of neck pain, flexion-extension views will be required before the patient's cervical spine can be considered cleared.

The CXR film shows a widened mediastinum, deviation of the nasogastric tube to the right, an indistinct aortic knob, and what appears to be either a left pleural effusion or left pulmonary contusion. These findings are consistent with an aortic arch injury. Such injuries occur as the result of high-speed deceleration and are associated with motor vehicle accidents or serious falls. Confirmation of the diagnosis of aortic arch injury requires an arch aortogram, which should be performed as soon as possible. Approximately 90% of patients sustaining such

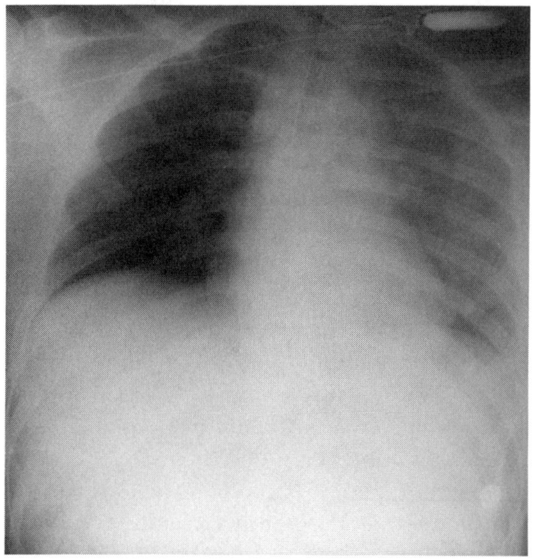

FIG 3-1

injuries are dead at the scene of the accident, and those surviving to reach the emergency department are at extremely high risk of free rupture of the aorta within the first few hours of hospitalization.

Reevaluation of the patient revealed that his HR had again climbed to the 130s and BP had fallen to 90/50. Breath sounds remained symmetrical. The abdomen remained mildly tender with voluntary guarding but was not significantly distended. Laboratory values returned to initial levels, and the patient's hematocrit was 24 with an Hb of 8.1 g/dl. ABG analysis demonstrated a pH of 7.21, partial pressure of carbon dioxide ($PCO_2$) of 30, and partial pressure of oxygen ($PO_2$) of 158 with 50% oxygen administered by face mask.

- *What is your assessment and plan at this point?*

This patient remained hemodynamically unstable with recurrent hypotension and tachycardia, a hematocrit of 24, and an arterial pH of 7.21 despite a $PCO_2$ of 30. These findings are consistent with hemorrhagic shock. The fact that this patient had already received 4 L of crystalloid and remained hypotensive suggests the possibility of ongoing bleeding. Although a significant injury of the aortic arch was suspected, it is important to remember that such injuries are rarely (if ever) the cause of gradually falling blood pressure. If the aorta should freely rupture into the pleural space, exsanguinating hemorrhage and death would occur within seconds. Therefore it is appropriate to consider other treatable causes of hypotension in this patient.

In addition, it is appropriate to increase the intensity of resuscitative efforts. The fact that this patient received 4 L of crystalloid and remained hypotensive can be considered an indication for the transfusion of O-negative or type-specific blood, if crossmatched blood is not yet available. It is important to remember that young, healthy patients have a tremendous ability to compensate for such hemorrhage, and although the patient remained alert and with a blood pressure of 90, this patient was in serious trouble and required continued aggressive support.

Potential sources of the ongoing bleeding included the presumed fractures of the left femur and left forearm. Such a fracture of the femur can easily be responsible for 2 to 4 units of blood loss, and the fracture of the forearm can account for an additional 1 to 2 units of blood loss. Pelvic fractures also can be responsible for extensive blood loss, and based on the initial physical examination, an anteroposterior film of the pelvis should be obtained. Finally, bleeding into the abdominal cavity should be seriously considered. This patient has obviously sustained a high-impact injury with risk of fracture of solid organs.

> An anteroposterior x-ray film of the pelvis was obtained (Fig. 3-2). X-ray films of the femur and left forearm confirmed compound, comminuted fractures in both extremities.
>
> ▪ *How would you proceed at this point?*

Once serious extremity fractures have been confirmed, the extremities should be immobilized until definitive therapy can be provided.

The x-ray film of the pelvis shows a marked diastasis of the pubic symphysis with fractures of the right pubic rami and left acetabulum and separation of the right sacroiliac joint. This "open book" type of fracture is often associated with extensive hemorrhage and could well contribute to the patient's ongoing hemodynamic instability. The options for management of this fracture, for the purposes of controlling bleeding, include placement of a pneumatic antishock garment, external fixation, and, if these methods are unsuccessful, angiography both for localization of the bleeding sites and possibly for angiographic embolization in an effort to control the bleeding. Military antishock trousers (MAST) are contraindicated in the setting of chest injuries, particularly in this case, in which increased BP in the chest resulting from inflation of the MAST may potentiate free rupture of the aorta.

> The patient was treated in the emergency department with external fixation of the pelvis for fracture stabilization and control of bleeding. After transfusion of 6 units of crossmatched blood and 4 units of fresh frozen plasma, the hemodynamic instability seemed to be largely controlled.
>
> The angiography team arrived and called for the patient. Potential intra-abdominal hemorrhage had not yet been ruled out, and although the patient was hemodynamically stable, the combination of the mechanism of injury, a history of hemodynamic instability, and a suspicious abdominal examination warrants further evaluation.
>
> ▪ *How would you proceed from here?*

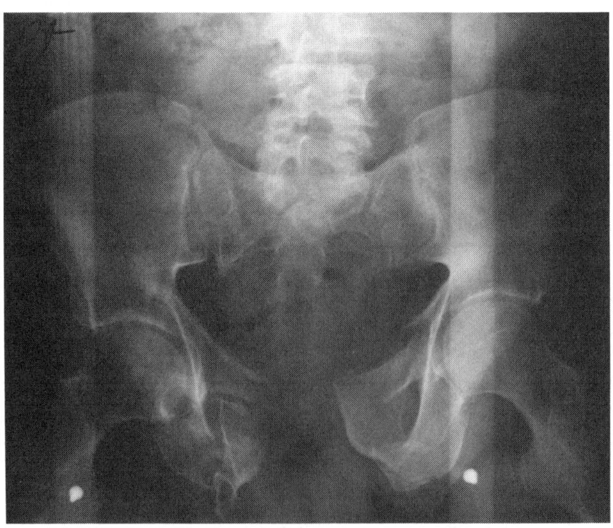

FIG 3-2

Options for evaluation of the abdomen include abdominal CT scan and diagnostic peritoneal lavage. Because it is critical to obtain the arch aortogram as soon as possible so that an injury to the aortic arch can be repaired if necessary, evaluation of other injuries should be done immediately. This would appear to be the ideal situation for use of diagnostic peritoneal lavage. With known pelvic fractures, the lavage should be performed via a supraumbilical approach in an effort to avoid retroperitoneal hematoma extending up from the pelvic fracture. The diagnostic accuracy of peritoneal lavage should exceed 95%, with a 2% to 3% false positive rate.

A diagnostic peritoneal lavage was performed via a supraumbilical approach. One thousand ml of lactated Ringer's solution was infused, and 800 ml of lavage fluid was returned. Although the lavage fluid appeared pink, the cell count revealed 40,000 RBC/mm$^3$ and 150 WBC/mm$^3$. Gram's stain showed no bacteria or food particles. No bile was detected.

- *How would you proceed from here?*

The diagnostic peritoneal lavage did not confirm significant abdominal injury. In the setting of blunt trauma, a positive lavage would be indicated by >100,000 RBC/mm$^3$ or >500 WBC/mm$^3$. Although there must be concern about the adequacy of the lavage, particularly in the setting of a retroperitoneal hematoma, the fact that 80% of the lavage fluid was returned without difficulty suggests an adequate test. At this point, the injury with highest priority is the suspected injury to the aortic arch.

The patient was taken to the angiography suite and the arch aortogram obtained (Fig. 3-3).

- *What is your plan of action?*

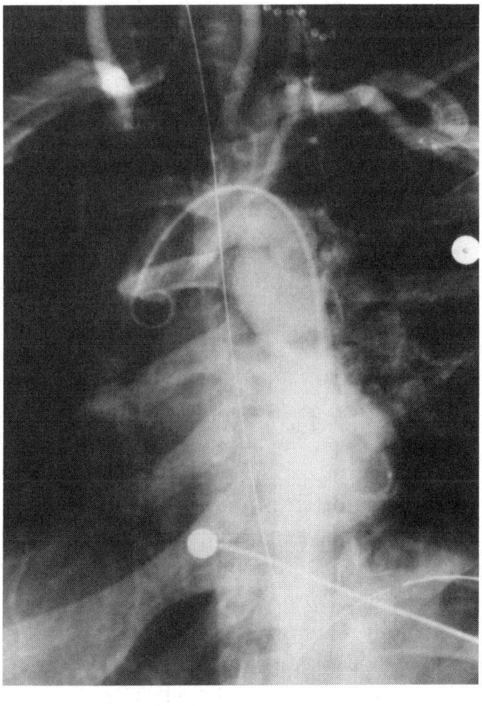

FIG 3-3

The arch aortogram shows a large pseudoaneurysm of the descending aorta just distal to the origin of the left subclavian artery. The patient should be taken directly to the operating room for exploration through a left thoracotomy incision for resection and placement of an aortic interposition graft to repair the traumatic dissection. Prior to leaving the operating room, the patient should undergo irrigation and debridement of the open fractures of the forearm and femur, both of which can be stabilized with external fixation. Placement of a suprapubic bladder catheter will be required if retrograde urethrogram confirms a urethral injury. Repair of the urethral injury is usually done 4 to 6 weeks after the initial injury.

At this point, the patient should be returned to the SICU for further resuscitation, until his acidosis and coagulopathy are controlled. He can return to the operating room for definitive repair of the extremity fractures and, if necessary, the pelvic fracture at a later date.

## CASE 2

A 59-year-old man was admitted to the emergency department after having been ejected from his pickup truck in a high-speed rollover. The patient apparently lost consciousness at the scene but was awake, with a Glasgow Coma Scale score of 13, when the paramedic personnel arrived. The patient complained of neck, chest, and abdominal pain and was mildly short of breath at the scene. He was transported by ambulance to the emergency department.

On arrival, the patient's BP was 130/90, HR was 115, and RR was 20. The chest wall was tender to anterior and lateral compression, particularly on the left side. Breath sounds were present in both hemithoraces but mildly decreased on the left side. On abdominal examination, bowel sounds were present, and there was a bruit heard over the umbilicus. The abdomen was not distended but was somewhat tender in the left upper quadrant. The patient was able to move all extremities. Dorsalis pedis and posterior tibial pulses were normal in the left lower extremity. In the right lower extremity, the dorsalis pedis pulse was not palpable, and the posterior tibial pulse was faint. A lateral cervical spine x-ray film and a portable CXR film were obtained and sent for development. Routine laboratory tests, including a urinalysis, were sent.

Before the x-ray films were returned, the patient became progressively short of breath, tachycardic, and tachypneic, with an RR of 30. BP fell to 80/40. At this point, the chest and cervical spine x-ray films were brought to the emergency department (Figs. 3-4 and 3-5).

- *What is your assessment and the appropriate course of action at this time?*

The CXR film shows an obvious tension pneumothorax with an air-filled left hemithorax and deviation of the heart and mediastinum into the right chest. If the physical examination had been repeated, breath sounds in the left chest would have been much more distant than on the initial examination and the trachea may have been deviated to the right side. The appropriate treatment at this point is placement of a chest tube, although if the patient deteriorates rapidly before a chest tube can be placed, a 14-gauge angiocatheter could be inserted into the left anterior chest at the midclavicular line at approximately the second or third intercostal space to temporarily relieve the tension pneumothorax.

The cervical spine film shows a severe fracture dislocation of the second and third vertebral bodies. It is unusual for a patient with such a severe fracture to be neurologically intact. This patient obviously should remain supported in a hard cervical collar until definitive treatment, such as Gardner-Wells tong traction or operative fixation, can be performed. In addition to a hard cervical collar, a firm backboard should be used to keep the patient immobilized. The head, neck, and torso can be secured to the backboard with straps or 2-inch tape for more secure immobilization.

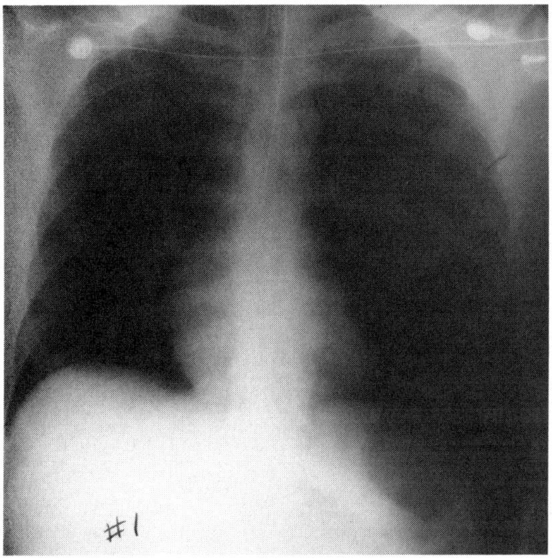

FIG 3-4

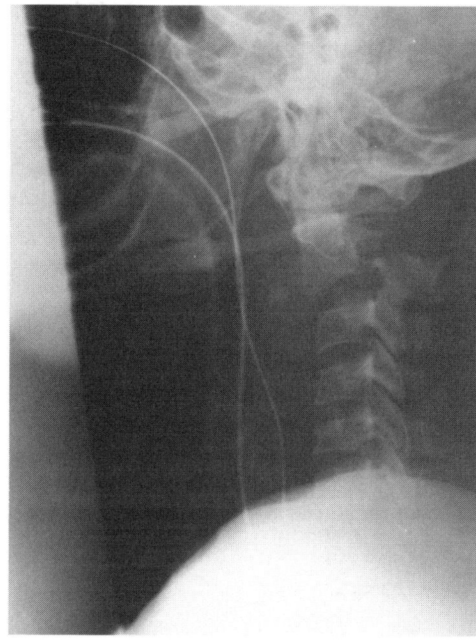

FIG 3-5

A left chest tube was placed through the anterior axillary line at the level of the inframammary crease with a large rush of air and instantaneous improvement in the patient's blood pressure and heart rate. Despite the improvement in his vital signs, however, the patient remained extremely short of breath. His respirations appeared labored, and on closer examination, his chest wall movements were somewhat discoordinant. A follow-up CXR film showed resolution of the tension pneumothorax; however, more careful examination of the film revealed multiple bilateral rib fractures.

- *What is the appropriate intervention at this point?*

The combination of multiple bilateral rib fractures and respiratory difficulty with discoordinant chest wall motion on respiration is consistent with the diagnosis of flail chest. Appropriate management at this point would be intubation and positive pressure mechanical ventilation. Unfortunately, the need to intubate this patient is complicated by the fracture of the cervical spine noted previously. Although orotracheal intubation (OTI) under direct visualization is the most reliable method of intubation, OTI is contraindicated under all but the most extreme circumstances when there is fracture of the cervical spine. A blind nasotracheal intubation (NTI) would be appropriate if there are no midfacial or basilar skull fractures. If such fractures were present, then surgical cricothyrotomy would be the procedure of choice to establish airway access.

Several attempts at blind NTI were made without success. In the setting of progressive respiratory distress, a surgical cricothyrotomy was performed. This procedure was done without difficulty, and a No. 6 cuffed tracheostomy tube was inserted.

At this juncture, results of the laboratory tests were returned. The hematocrit was 31.5, WBC count was 15,000/$mm^3$, electrolytes and creatinine levels were normal, and a urinalysis demonstrated 50 to 100 RBC/$mm^3$

- *What is your assessment at this time?*

Although this patient had been hemodynamically stable, a hematocrit of 31.5 suggests undiagnosed hemorrhage. The elevated WBC count, although usually regarded as suggestive of infection, is a normal response to stress and injury and in this case may not be significant. Diagnosing the source of blood loss in this patient should not be particularly difficult. He had no apparent extremity fractures, and his pelvis was stable on initial examination. The CXR film did not suggest blood loss into the chest, and, by the process of elimination, unexplained blood loss into the abdominal cavity must be considered. Although the patient's abdomen was not distended and a surgical abdomen was not obvious, the patient did complain of pain and tenderness in the left upper abdominal quadrant; therefore further evaluation of the abdomen is indicated.

Appropriate diagnostic procedures would include a diagnostic peritoneal lavage, by either open or closed technique, or an abdominal CT scan. Both studies are reliable and should yield a diagnosis in 95% of cases. The advantage of peritoneal lavage is that it can be performed rapidly and inexpensively. The abdominal CT scan requires more time and costs more, but it can be used to assess retroperitoneal structures, such as the duodenum, pancreas, and kidneys. Because this patient remains hemodynamically stable, and time is therefore less important, and because of the 50 to 100 RBC/mm$^3$ on urinalysis, an abdominal CT scan would be my favored procedure. Certainly the clinician could not be faulted for obtaining a diagnostic peritoneal lavage to evaluate the peritoneal cavity, followed by an intravenous pyelogram and cystogram to evaluate the hematuria.

> An abdominal CT scan was obtained (Fig. 3-6). While in the CT scanner, the patient seemed somewhat agitated, and on further questioning, it became clear that he was complaining of pain in the right lower extremity. Examination of the right lower extremity revealed that distal pulses were absent. The extremity was cold, and the patient was unable to move it.
>
> - *What is your assessment and your plan of action at this point?*

The abdominal CT scan shows a splenic laceration and a fairly large perisplenic hematoma. Other CT scan cuts, not shown here, showed a moderate amount of blood within the peritoneal cavity; intact kidneys, collecting systems, and ureters bilaterally; no extravasation of contrast from the bladder; no obvious abnormality in the aorta or iliac arteries; and no apparent pelvic

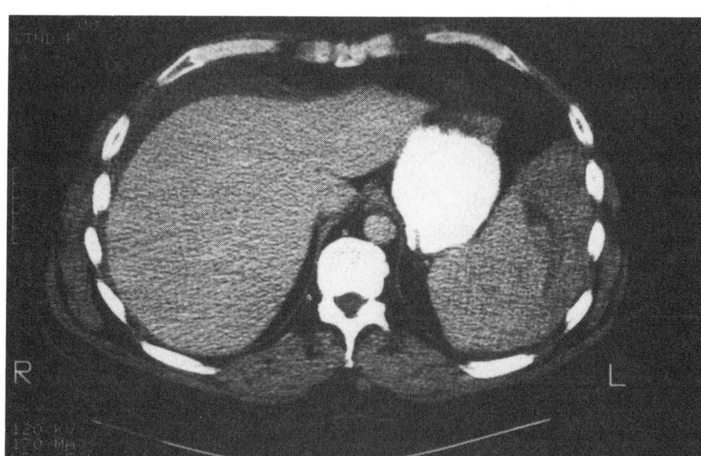


FIG 3-6

fracture. Management of the splenic injury depends on the clinical situation. Laparotomy for splenectomy or possible splenic repair is always appropriate in this situation, but some clinicians might choose to observe the splenic injury by admitting the patient to the SICU for evaluation with serial hematocrits, abdominal examinations, and a repeat CT scan in 24 hours. When multiple injuries are present, which may complicate the nonsurgical management of the splenic injury, laparotomy is probably the management method of choice.

The decision was made to take the patient to the operating room for his splenic injury, although the patient's right lower extremity remained something of a mystery. His inability to move the extremity raised the question of spinal cord injury, particularly in the presence of a known fracture of the cervical spine; however, the fact that the extremity was cold and pulseless indicated the possibility of arterial injury. Although no aortic or iliac artery injury was recognized on abdominal CT scan, the fact remained that this patient had no femoral, popliteal, or distal pulses in the right lower extremity. The absence of a femoral pulse is consistent with an arterial obstruction proximally.

- *What is the appropriate course of action at this point?*

Because plans had been made to take the patient to the operating room for his splenic injury, some clinicians would argue that exploration of the aorta and iliac vessels at surgery would be appropriate management of the suspected arterial injury. On the other hand, angiography might be extremely helpful in delineating the location and extent of the arterial injury. Because the patient was hemodynamically stable and was admitted with a normal creatinine concentration, there are no contraindications to the performance of angiography. The patient already had an abdomimal CT scan with contrast enhancement, and therefore the dye load for the anticipated angiogram should be minimized.

An aortogram of the distal aorta was obtained (Fig. 3-7). Note the occlusion of the right common iliac artery at the aortic bifurcation with a small intimal flap protruding over the

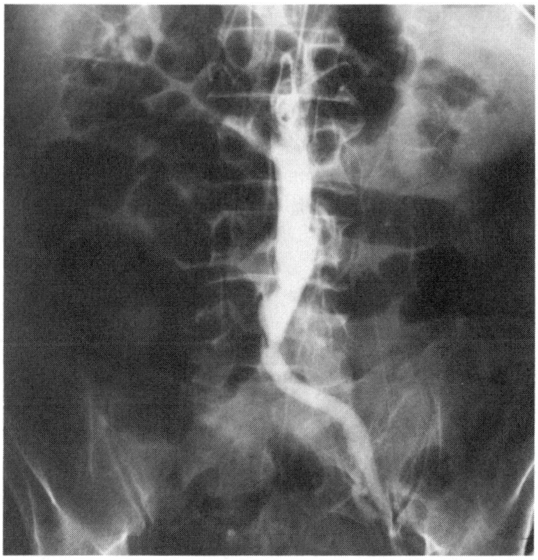

FIG 3-7

orifice to the left common iliac artery. There is a pseudoaneurysm extending proximally to the level of the inferior mesenteric artery.

- *What is your plan of action at this point?*

This patient obviously sustained a severe injury to the distal aorta with occlusion of the right common iliac artery and threatened occlusion of the left common iliac artery. Although injuries to the distal aorta are unusual, this angiogram offers evidence that such injuries do indeed occur. The mechanism of injury is probably direct compression of the aorta resulting from direct blunt impact. The patient should be taken to the operating room for exploratory laparotomy and exploration of the distal aorta. Remember that the limit to warm ischemia in a devascularized extremity is 4 to 6 hours, so repair should be accomplished as soon as possible. The presence of this aortic injury makes exploration mandatory. Both the splenic injury and the aortic injuries can be dealt with at exploratory laparotomy.

Because the aortic repair may require heparin anticoagulation, the possibility of intracerebral hemorrhage is significant. This patient sustained a significant loss of consciousness at the scene of the accident and had a mildly depressed mental status on arrival at the emergency department. These findings alone are sufficient to warrant a CT scan of the head. In anticipation of a prolonged surgical procedure that may require anticoagulation, the CT scan should be obtained prior to surgery.

A CT scan of the head without contrast enhancement showed no evidence of intracerebral or extra-axial hemorrhage.

The patient was taken to the operating room, where he was found to have a splenic laceration with approximately 700 ml of blood within the peritoneal cavity. Although the laceration was not actively bleeding, the presence of another serious injury mandated splenectomy. The procedure was done without difficulty. Exploration of the distal aorta revealed a pseudoaneurysm extending from the inferior mesenteric artery to the aortic bifurcation. After proximal and distal control were obtained, the distal aorta was opened. An extensive dissection and pseudoaneurysm within the distal aorta precluded an endarterectomy, and therefore the injury was treated with an interposition aortic graft. Care was taken to tack the intima of the iliac artery to the remainder of the arterial wall. Fogarty embolectomy was performed on the right iliac and femoral system to restore blood flow to the right lower extremity.

The patient tolerated the surgical procedure without difficulty and was then transported to the SICU. His cervical spine fracture could initially be managed with Gardner-Wells tong traction until he was stable from a hemodynamic and respiratory standpoint, at which time he would be treated by placement of a halo brace for long-term management. The patient remained neurologically intact. He will likely require prolonged mechanical ventilation for his chest injuries and a prolonged stay in the hospital rehabilitation unit after extubation.

# CHAPTER 4

# *Cardiovascular Risk: Assessment and Reduction*

Jon F. Berlauk

## CASE 1

An 86-year-old woman was admitted to the SICU for a "tune-up" prior to vascular surgery. She was disabled because of a nonhealing ulcer and ischemic toes on the left foot. The ulcer had been treated with topical dressings and parenteral antibiotics for several months without improvement. Recently, the patient's foot had become painful at rest. A femoral artery to distal limb bypass using an in situ vein graft was planned for the next morning.

The patient gave a history of diabetes mellitus for 44 years, treated with insulin in recent years. Complications of her disease included retinal blindness for 25 years, renal insufficiency, and severe peripheral vascular disease. She had had hypertension for 20 years as well as angina in recent years, but there was no history of previous myocardial infarction, congestive heart failure, or cerebrovascular accident. Her medication included neutral protamine Hagedorn (NPH) insulin 11 units subcutaneously every morning, diuretic/antihypertensive (e.g., Dyazide) one tablet daily, isosorbide dinitrate 10 mg qid, amitriptyline 50 mg, and pentazocine at bedtime.

Physical examination revealed a frail, pleasant woman lying in bed. She had a gauze dressing on her left foot. Auscultation of the heart and lungs was normal. The most conspicuous physical findings were in the lower extremities. The patient had no palpable pulses below the knees bilaterally. The left foot was cool to the touch but had normal sensation and movement. The toes appeared dusky blue, and a large ulcer was present over the left medial malleolus.

Blood chemistry analyses gave the following values:

| Na | K | Cl | $HCO_3^-$ | BUN | Cr | Hb |
|---|---|---|---|---|---|---|
| 141 | 4.1 | 106 | 26 | 29 | 1.7 | 10.6 |

The CXR results were within normal limits. An ECG showed normal sinus rhythm with a small Q wave in lead III.

This patient's preoperative risk factors included old age, angina, diabetes mellitus, hypertension, and peripheral vascular disease. Computation of cardiac risk index (CRI) would place her in class II with 8 points (age >70 years = 5; bedridden status = 3); thus her estimated risk for major complications would be 7% to 11%. This seems appropriate, given her condition

This chapter can be studied in conjunction with *Essentials of Surgical Critical Care,* edited by Jerome H. Abrams and Frank B. Cerra (St. Louis: Quality Medical Publishing, Inc., 1993), Chapter 6.

and the anticipated stress of the surgical procedure. The patient's history of angina is troublesome, however. Her exercise tolerance is unknown because of her disability. Laboratory stress testing might prove helpful in determining the severity of her coronary artery disease (CAD), but would she want a coronary artery bypass graft (CABG) or percutaneous transluminal coronary angioplasty (PTCA) if the results of testing led to that decision? Would a CABG (or PTCA) prior to vascular surgery reduce her overall morbidity and mortality risk? Do you even need further information about her coronary anatomy? Can intensive perioperative medical care alone reduce her risk? These questions should be addressed for every high-risk surgical patient. The answers will not always fit an algorithm.

The patient did not want to undergo a CABG, so no further diagnostic tests were ordered. After a pulmonary artery (PA) catheter and a radial artery catheter had been placed, the following baseline cardiovascular values were obtained:

*Measured variables*

| BP | HR | CO | PA | CVP | PCWP |
|---|---|---|---|---|---|
| 197/79 | 97 | 4.6 | 50/24 | 9 | 21 |

*Derived variables*

| CI | SV | SVR | PVR |
|---|---|---|---|
| 2.7 | 48 | 1901 | 203 |

- *What is your interpretation? What would you do next?*

You may wonder if the elevated BP and HR truly reflect baseline physiologic status. The stress associated with insertion of invasive catheters is significant.[1] Adequate intravenous and subcutaneous anesthesia are mandatory, especially in a patient with significant ischemic heart disease. Despite these concerns, the patient's cardiac index (CI) is relatively low even with the elevated HR. Her systemic vascular resistance (SVR) is also high. This combination alone could reflect acute and chronic hypertensive physiologic conditions. However, her PCWP also is elevated. This is a surprising finding since the patient had no signs or symptoms of congestive heart failure. One interpretation could be acute left ventricular dysfunction because of ischemia. Another reasonable interpretation would be chronic left ventricular dysfunction secondary to diabetic cardiomyopathy. Either also would explain her low CI and elevated SVR. Note the poor correlation between CVP and PCWP.

One inch of nitropaste was applied to the chest wall. After 30 minutes the PCWP was remeasured and still found to be elevated. No fluid was administered. Sodium nitroprusside (SNP) was titrated to a 1 mg/kg/min infusion. To keep the BP >120 systolic, 600 ml of crystalloid was administered. After an appropriate time the cardiovascular profile was repeated:

*Measured variables*

| BP | HR | CO | PA | CVP | PCWP |
|---|---|---|---|---|---|
| 144/56 | 99 | 5.3 | 36/15 | 8 | 12 |

*Derived variables*

| CI | SV | SVR | PVR |
|---|---|---|---|
| 3.1 | 54 | 1152 | 151 |

- *What is your interpretation?*

The patient's left ventricular dysfunction did not seem to be an acute (ischemic) problem. Therefore pharmacologic intervention to improve myocardial performance was appropriate. Either positive inotropic agents or afterload-reducing drugs will improve cardiac performance. If the BP and SVR are elevated, I generally choose an afterload-reducing agent. SNP was chosen instead of nitroglycerin because it results in better afterload reduction. However, given the patient's history of angina, nitroglycerin may have been appropriate. Nevertheless, as a result of this intervention, her test results nearly met the major criteria for a successful cardiovascular tune-up. Her PCWP was between 8 and 15 mm Hg and her CI was >2.8 L/min/m$^2$. Only the SVR was slightly above the recommended 1100 dyne · sec · cm$^{-5}$. However, the HR was still elevated, and although the SV improved slightly, you may question whether overall myocardial performance was augmented.

Dopamine was started at 3 μg/kg/min to improve myocardial contractility. An additional 500 ml of crystalloid was carefully administered and the cardiovascular study was repeated:

*Measured variables*

| BP | HR | CO | PA | CVP | PCWP |
|---|---|---|---|---|---|
| 132/58 | 92 | 5.6 | 40/20 | 12 | 10 |

*Derived variables*

| CI | SV | SVR | PVR |
|---|---|---|---|
| 3.3 | 61 | 1014 | 243 |

At this point, the patient was judged to have optimal cardiovascular performance. Note the disparity between CVP and PCWP again. The CVP and PCWP have been found to correlate and trend together only if myocardial function is normal (left ventricular ejection fraction >50%).[2] With left ventricular dysfunction, the CVP not only correlates poorly with the PCWP, but also it may change in the opposite direction.

This patient underwent a successful operation without complication and was discharged from the hospital 9 days later.

## REFERENCES

1. Lunn JK, Stanley TH, Webster LR, et al. Arterial blood-pressure and pulse-rate responses to pulmonary and radial arterial catheterization prior to cardiac and major vascular operations. Anesthesiology 51:265, 1979.
2. Mangano DT. Monitoring pulmonary arterial pressure in coronary-artery disease. Anesthesiology 53:364, 1980.

## CASE 2

An 88-year-old man was sent to the SICU for a "tune-up" prior to an urgent cholecystectomy. He had been admitted to the hospital 2 days earlier with right upper quadrant abdominal pain and nausea. An abdominal ultrasound examination confirmed the presence of gallstones, but no biliary obstruction could be detected. The pain resolved but returned several hours later. A repeat ultrasound examination demonstrated a dilated, thick-walled gallbladder.

The patient gave a history of diabetes mellitus treated with insulin for 6 years. He had been hospitalized for heart failure 8 years before and was told he had atrial fibrillation. He denied angina or recent heart failure. He had had a femoropopliteal artery bypass 2 years earlier but currently exercised very little because of claudication in his left calf. The patient's medications included nifedipine 10 mg tid, furosemide 20 mg bid, potassium supplement 25 mEq tid, and digoxin 0.25 mg daily.

Physical examination revealed a thin, frail man who appeared comfortable. He had a slow, irregular pulse. Auscultation confirmed the irregular heart rhythm. The patient's lungs were clear. He had no jugular venous distention at 30-degree elevation. Examination of the abdomen revealed tenderness and guarding in the right upper quadrant. Bowel sounds were absent. The abdomen was tympanitic to percussion.

Blood chemistry analyses gave the following values:

| Na | K | Cl | $HCO_3^-$ | BUN | Cr | Hb |
|---|---|---|---|---|---|---|
| 135 | 4.3 | 98 | 31 | 31 | 1.2 | 14.7 |

A CXR film showed a tortuous aorta but clear lung fields. An ECG revealed atrial fibrillation and nonspecific ST-T changes consistent with digitalis.

This patient had the following preoperative risk factors: old age, diabetes mellitus, dysrhythmia, and peripheral vascular disease. He would receive 15 points on his CRI (old age = 5, dysrhythmia = 7, intraperitoneal operation = 3), placing him in class III. His risk for perioperative complications would be between 14% and 38%. In addition, the patient has a remote history of CHF. Clearly he deserves preoperative cardiovascular assessment, limited somewhat by the urgency of his cholecystitis.

After the appropriate catheters were placed, the following baseline cardiovascular values were obtained:

*Measured variables*

| BP | HR | CO | PA | CVP | PCWP |
|---|---|---|---|---|---|
| 156/70 | 58 | 3.5 | 27/18 | 2 | 9 |

*Derived variables*

| CI | SV | SVR | PVR |
|---|---|---|---|
| 1.8 | 60 | 2209 | 91 |

- *What is your interpretation? What would you do next?*

The patient had a high SVR, a remarkably low CI, but a normal PCWP. The cardiac output (CO) may be falsely low during any cardiac dysrhythmia, depending on the HR at the time of fluid injection.[1] However, this is usually caused by acute unstable rhythms, not stable dysrhythmias.[2] Nevertheless, if the CO were falsely low, the SVR would be falsely elevated. Excluding measurement errors, this profile is consistent with severe, chronic hypertension, but the patient denied a history of hypertension. In fact, his baseline BP is probably normal for his age. Alternatively, he may have chronic CHF and currently be dehydrated. This would be consistent with his clinical history as well as the laboratory findings. The patient's BUN/Cr ratio is elevated beyond 20, indicating a prerenal azotemia. His serum bicarbonate is elevated, suggesting metabolic alkalosis possibly induced by vomiting and/or diuretic therapy. Even his Hb may represent hemoconcentration. If the patient does have LVD, in the presence of intravascular volume depletion, his heart would not be functioning on the optimal portion of the Frank-Starling curve. His CI would be low despite the "normal" PCWP. A judicious fluid challenge would seem appropriate under any circumstance.

Nitropaste was applied to the patient's chest, and an infusion of 250 ml of hydroxyethyl starch was started. The PCWP rose from 9 to 10 mm Hg, and the CVP rose to 4 mm Hg during the 20-minute infusion. The patient's BP also climbed to 182/88; the HR remained at 58. After these values had been obtained, an infusion of nitroglycerin was started. An additional 250 ml of hydroxyethyl starch and 250 ml of crystalloid was administered as the nitroglycerin was titrated to 1.8 μg/kg/min. The following cardiovascular values were then obtained:

*Measured variables*

| BP | HR | CO | PA | CVP | PCWP |
|---|---|---|---|---|---|
| 150/70 | 70 | 4.6 | 25/12 | 2 | 8 |

*Derived variables*

| CI | SV | SVR | PVR |
|---|---|---|---|
| 2.3 | 66 | 1646 | 75 |

- *What is your interpretation?*

The patient responded normally to an initial fluid challenge. A patient with LVD would have demonstrated an abrupt rise in PCWP after a rapid fluid bolus. Instead of chronic CHF, the patient appears to have underlying hypertension and significant intravascular volume depletion. Despite the patient's response to a fluid challenge, his cardiovascular physiologic condition is worrisome. Although his left ventricular function is reasonable, it is not normal. Intravenous vasodilators are not necessary to improve blood flow in a patient with normal left ventricular function.

In an attempt to increase the CI and decrease the SVR, SNP was infused. Hydroxyethyl starch 250 ml and crystalloid 500 ml were administered as the SNP was titrated to 0.9 μg/kg/min. A repeat cardiovascular study revealed:

*Measured variables*

| BP | HR | CO | PA | CVP | PCWP |
|---|---|---|---|---|---|
| 136/64 | 70 | 6.4 | 32/14 | 8 | 9 |

*Derived variables*

| CI | SV | SVR | PVR |
|---|---|---|---|
| 3.2 | 91 | 983 | 138 |

At this point the patient was judged to have an optimum cardiovascular physiologic state and was taken to the operating room. He underwent an uneventful cholecystectomy and was discharged from the hospital 6 days later.

## REFERENCES

1. Harris AP, Miller CF, Beattie C, et al. The slowing of sinus rhythm during thermodilution cardiac output determination and the effect of altering injectate temperature. Anesthesiology 63:540, 1985.
2. Todd MM. Atrial fibrillation induced by the right atrial injection of cold fluids during thermodilution cardiac output determination: A case report. Anesthesiology 59:253, 1983.

## CASE 3

A 73-year-old woman was admitted to the hospital with a nonhealing ulcer on the right great toe. She had had severe peripheral vascular disease for many years, which required a left femoroanterior tibial artery bypass 5 years previously and amputations of the second and third toes of the right foot 5 months ago. The ulcer developed shortly after the toe amputations, and the patient responded poorly to the conservative therapy provided by her nursing home. She was scheduled for a right in situ vein graft bypass for foot salvage. In preparation, she was sent to the SICU for a "tune-up."

The patient's history included two cerebrovascular accidents several years earlier. She recovered nearly all of her motor function on both occasions but suffered mental deterioration. She had had congestive heart failure precipitated by atrial fibrillation 4 years before and had had intermittent episodes of orthopnea, paroxysmal nocturnal dyspnea, and dyspnea with mild exertion in the recent past. She slept on three pillows. The patient had had hypertension for 14 years but denied diabetes mellitus, angina, or myocardial infarction. In addition, she had gout and osteoarthritis currently under good control. Her medications included furosemide 80 mg bid, potassium chloride (e.g., Slow-K) 2 tablets daily, naproxen 375 mg bid, hydralazine 50 mg bid, allopurinol 300 mg daily, warfarin 2.5 mg every other day, and Tylenol No. 3 as needed for foot pain.

Physical examination showed an overweight woman who appeared ill. Neurologic examination revealed only mild weakness of the left arm. Bibasilar rales could be heard on auscultation. Also, a grade III/VI systolic ejection murmur radiating to the carotids was heard as well as a second holosystolic murmur that was loudest at the apex of the heart. There was a questionable $S_3$ gallop. The patient had diminished pulses in both lower extremities, a necrotic ulcer on the right great toe, and bilateral marked skin changes of stasis dermatitis.

Blood chemistry analyses gave the following values:

| Na | K | Cl | $HCO_3^-$ | BUN | Cr | Hb |
|---|---|---|---|---|---|---|
| 144 | 4.6 | 102 | 33 | 42 | 1.3 | 12.3 |

A CXR film showed cardiomegaly with increased pulmonary vascular marking and a small left pleural effusion. An ECG revealed left ventricular hypertrophy (LVH) with repolarization changes, atrial fibrillation, and possible old anteroseptal MI. M-mode and two-dimensional ultrasound cardiography showed concentric LVH and marked left atrial enlargement with significant mitral insufficiency. The aortic valve was thickened but functioned adequately. Moderate pericardial effusion was apparent.

This patient was at serious risk for perioperative cardiac complications. Her historical risk factors included severe peripheral vascular disease, congestive heart failure, hypertension, dysrhythmia, cerebrovascular accident, valvular heart disease, and old age. In addition, cardiomegaly on CXR film and an abnormal ECG have been found to predict increased risk. Her CRI totaled 26 points, placing her in class IV. The accompanying risk for major complications would be estimated at greater than 30%. She could easily have been considered an unacceptable surgical candidate from the information available thus far, but because her surgeon believed she would lose her foot without surgery, an attempt was made to optimize her cardiovascular function.

Invasive catheters were placed without complications, and the following baseline cardiovascular values were obtained:

*Measured variables*

| BP | HR | CO | PA | CVP | PCWP |
|---|---|---|---|---|---|
| 152/87 | 82 | 3.4 | 70/39 | 15 | 30 |

*Derived variables*

| CI | SV | SVR | PVR |
|---|---|---|---|
| 2.1 | 41 | 2204 | 243 |

- *What is your interpretation?*

It should not be surprising that this patient had an elevated PCWP, low cardiac output, and elevated SVR. The question is whether she would improve with pharmacologic intervention.

No fluid was given because of the elevated PCWP. A nitroglycerin infusion was started and titrated to 1 μg/kg/min. The cardiovascular study was repeated:

*Measured variables*

| BP | HR | CO | PA | CVP | PCWP |
|---|---|---|---|---|---|
| 154/77 | 102 | 4.0 | 50/22 | 12 | 18 |

*Derived variables*

| CI | SV | SVR | PVR |
|---|---|---|---|
| 2.5 | 39 | 1813 | 186 |

Nitroglycerin was slowly increased to 2 μg/kg/min while 200 ml of plasma was infused over 2 hours. Four hours after the initial cardiovascular studies, the profile was:

*Measured variables*

| BP | HR | CO | PA | CVP | PCWP |
|---|---|---|---|---|---|
| 133/64 | 111 | 5.3 | 65/35 | 13 | 26 |

*Derived variables*

| CI | SV | SVR | PVR |
|---|---|---|---|
| 3.2 | 48 | 1117 | 151 |

- *Is the patient ready for surgery?*

Despite the apparent improvement in the patient's CI, most of the change can be attributed to an increase in HR. Her SV remained relatively unchanged. The persistently elevated PCWP is worrisome. The patient did not appear to be significantly improved. Indeed, auscultation of her chest revealed increased rales to the midlung fields despite the fact that her total intake/output was 520 ml/530 ml to this point. Surgery was postponed after a discussion of these findings with the surgeon. The plan was to give her digitalis and intravenous inotropes for another 24 hours, then reassess her condition.

Digitalis 0.25 mg was given intravenously and repeated 4 and 8 hours later. A dobutamine infusion was begun. Eight hours later nitroglycerin was infused at 6 μg/kg/min and dobutamine at 2.5 μg/kg/min. The following cardiovascular values were obtained:

*Measured variables*

| BP | HR | CO | PA | CVP | PCWP |
|---|---|---|---|---|---|
| 162/70 | 96 | 4.3 | 60/32 | 11 | 22 |

*Derived variables*

| CI | SV | SVR | PVR |
|---|---|---|---|
| 2.7 | 44 | 1668 | 174 |

An arteriovenous oxygen content (A-$Vo_2$) difference was measured at 7 vol%. Intravenous nitroglycerin was discontinued and SNP was begun. Two hours later, with dobutamine infusing at 5 μg/kg/min and SNP at 2 μg/kg/min, the cardiovascular values were:

*Measured variables*

| BP | HR | CO | PA | CVP | PCWP |
|---|---|---|---|---|---|
| 145/67 | 110 | 5.3 | 58/37 | 12 | 29 |

*Derived variables*

| CI | SV | SVR | PVR |
|---|---|---|---|
| 3.2 | 48 | 1223 | 106 |

SNP was increased to 3.1 μg/kg/min over the next 6 hours; the dobutamine remained at 5 μg/kg/min. The following cardiovascular values were obtained:

*Measured variables*

| BP | HR | CO | PA | CVP | PCWP |
|---|---|---|---|---|---|
| 138/64 | 118 | 5.7 | 65/38 | 17 | 29 |

*Derived variables*

| CI | SV | SVR | PVR |
|---|---|---|---|
| 3.6 | 48 | 804 | 210 |

- *What is your evaluation?*

The combination of a positive inotropic agent and an afterload-reducing drug usually will augment cardiac performance in a patient with congestive heart failure.[1] However, some elderly patients have uncorrectable cardiovascular pathophysiology.[2] This patient is a case in point. Her "improved" CI is still a function of heart rate and not improved cardiac performance. Her PCWP is essentially unchanged after 24 hours of intensive pharmacologic intervention.

The patient still had bibasilar rales on auscultation. Her intake/output for the previous 24 hours was 1140 ml/1220 ml. High-dose intravenous furosemide and bumetanide produced only a 400-ml urine output over the next 8 hours. The dobutamine infusion was at 2.5 μg/kg/min and SNP was at 3.6 μg/kg/min when the last cardiovascular study was made:

*Measured variables*

| BP | HR | CO | PA | CVP | PCWP |
|---|---|---|---|---|---|
| 168/59 | 99 | 5.1 | 72/39 | 17 | 30 |

*Derived variables*

| CI | SV | SVR | PVR |
|---|---|---|---|
| 3.1 | 52 | 967 | 173 |

The A-$VO_2$ difference was now 5.2 vol%. The patient's surgery was cancelled and further conservative therapy continued. She improved sufficiently to be discharged back to her nursing home 28 days later.

## REFERENCES

1. Miller RR, Awan NA, Joye JA, et al. Combined dopamine and nitroprusside therapy in congestive heart failure. Greater augmentation of cardiac performance by addition of inotropic stimulation to afterload reduction. Circulation 55:881, 1977.
2. Del Guercio LRM, Cohn JD. Monitoring operative risk in the elderly. JAMA 243:1350, 1980.

## CASE 4

A 63-year-old woman was transferred to the SICU for a "tune-up" prior to lower extremity vascular surgery. She had been admitted to the hospital because of a nonhealing ulcer on her left great toe. She was having increasing difficulty walking because of the ulcer and left calf claudication. An in situ vein graft bypass procedure was planned.

The patient had a 10-year history of diabetes mellitus that was treated only with dietary restriction. Three years earlier she had had a four-vessel coronary artery bypass graft after an episode of congestive heart failure. She denied a history of angina, myocardial infarction, or cerebrovascular accident but did admit to hypertension for at least 20 years. She denied recent symptoms of congestive heart failure.

Her medications included bumetanide 1 mg bid, digoxin 0.25 mg daily, and captopril 25 mg bid.

Physical examination showed a well-nourished woman with a bandaged left foot. She had no jugular venous distention at 30-degree elevation. Auscultation of her heart revealed a grade III/VI holosystolic murmur radiating to the axilla. The patient's lung fields were clear to auscultation. The left leg had surgical scars from her previous vein harvesting for the coronary artery bypass graft (CABG). There were no palpable pulses below the knee. A small ulcer was present on the lateral left great toe.

Blood chemistry analyses gave the following values:

| Na | K | Cl | $HCO_3^-$ | BUN | Cr | Hb |
|---|---|---|---|---|---|---|
| 136 | 5.3 | 102 | 29 | 16 | 1.0 | 13.5 |

A CXR film showed surgical clips and sternal wires from her prior CABG, but otherwise findings were within normal limits. An ECG showed normal sinus rhythm with nonspecific ST-T changes consistent with digitalis.

A cardiology consultation was obtained shortly after the patient's admission to the hospital. The cardiologist found "no objective evidence for ischemic heart disease" presently, but her "functional status made it difficult to evaluate." An ultrasound cardiogram showed "lateral wall motion abnormality which could be 2° to MI," but overall her "ventricular function was not grossly impaired." She was considered an acceptable risk for the anticipated surgery.

This patient had several historical predictors of perioperative complications including hypertension, diabetes mellitus, peripheral vascular disease, and previous CABG. The CABG is the most interesting among them. Several studies confirm that a previous CABG protects a patient from a postoperative myocardial infarction. The incidence of postoperative myocardial infarction in patients with a prior CABG is 0% to 1.2% versus 1.1% to 6% in patients without a previous CABG; the mortality rate is 0.5% to 0.9% vs. 1% to 2.4%.[1] However, this protective benefit begins only 4 to 6 weeks following a CABG.[2] Since this patient's CABG was performed several years before, her risk would be diminished, provided that her coronary grafts were still functioning.

The cardiology consultation may sound reassuring, but the ultrasound cardiogram has not been found to be a reliable predictor of cardiac risk.[1] The CRI is more helpful despite its limitations. This patient's CRI score would place her in class I with an estimated 1% to 7% risk of major complications.

The invasive catheters were placed, and the following cardiovascular profile was obtained:

*Measured variables*

| BP | HR | CO | PA | CVP | PCWP |
|---|---|---|---|---|---|
| 192/86 | 101 | 5.2 | 50/28 | 4 | 8 |

*Derived variables*

| CI | SV | SVR | PVR |
|---|---|---|---|
| 3.2 | 51 | 1969 | 113 |

- *What is your interpretation?*

Upon casual analysis, this profile suggests a fairly normal patient with only a moderately elevated SVR. This abnormality could be explained by the high BP. The CI and PCWP look normal. A closer evaluation, however, would determine that the cardiac output is normal only because the HR is elevated. In addition, the PA pressure is abnormally high. One of the criteria for a valid PCWP is a PCWP less than the PA pressure, but this gradient between the PCWP and PA pressure seems excessive.

Because the PCWP was <15 mm Hg, 500 ml of hydroxyethyl starch was administered and nitropaste was applied to the chest wall. Two hours later the cardiovascular profile revealed:

*Measured variables*

| BP | HR | CO | PA | CVP | PCWP |
|---|---|---|---|---|---|
| 206/92 | 97 | 4.3 | 72/48 | 11 | >25 |

*Derived variables*

| CI | SV | SVR | PVR |
|---|---|---|---|
| 2.7 | 44 | 2288 | 484 |

The interpretation was that this patient had a noncompliant ventricle and could not tolerate fluid well. A nitroglycerin drip was started at 0.2 μg/kg/min. After 1 hour the following cardiovascular profile was obtained:

*Measured variables*

| BP | HR | CO | PA | CVP | PCWP |
|---|---|---|---|---|---|
| 193/80 | 91 | 5.5 | 54/30 | 7 | 10 |

*Derived variables*

| CI | SV | SVR | PVR |
|---|---|---|---|
| 3.1 | 60 | 1610 | 407 |

Since the PCWP was now "low" again, 500 ml of hydroxyethyl starch was ordered.

- *What is your evaluation? Would you be concerned about the persistently elevated HR and BP?*

A patient with a noncompliant left ventricle will indeed respond to an acute volume challenge with an increase in BP, PCWP, and perhaps a decrease in CI. However, if the PCWP is "normal," you would expect the PA pressure to be normal as well. Given time, the patient will redistribute the fluid, and the cardiovascular variables will shift back toward baseline measurements. This patient did not redistribute the initial 500 ml of colloid after 2 hours and yet was seemingly "cured" with an unimpressive dose of nitroglycerin. Something is not right. Finally, a persistently elevated HR and BP is of great concern in any patient with cardiac disease.

The 500 ml of colloid was infused over 2 hours, and the nitroglycerin was increased to 0.5 μg/kg/min. Three hours after the last study, the following cardiovascular profile was obtained:

*Measured variables*

| BP | HR | CO | PA | CVP | PCWP |
|---|---|---|---|---|---|
| 180/80 | 92 | 4.7 | 75/44 | 9 | 32 |

*Derived variables*

| CI | SV | SVR | PVR |
|---|---|---|---|
| 3 | 51 | 1776 | 380 |

The A-$Vo_2$ difference was 7.5 vol%.

By now it seems apparent that this cardiovascular profile reflects the true pathophysiologic condition of the patient. The interpretation of the baseline profile was wrong because too much emphasis was placed on a single measurement, the PCWP.

No further fluids were given because of the elevated PCWP. The nitroglycerin drip was continued at 0.5 μg/kg/min. At about 1 hour after the last study, the patient complained of chest "fullness and pressure" extending into her left arm. Oxygen administered by nasal cannula was started. The ABG data were 7.39/41/65/25 on oxygen 6 L/min. An ECG showed new ST-segment depression in leads $V_2$ through $V_6$. A CXR film showed increased pulmonary vasculature consistent with pulmonary edema. Surgery was cancelled, and a cardiology consultation was obtained. The cardiologist agreed that surgery should be postponed until myocardial infarction was ruled out. The creatine phosphokinase (CPK-MB) measured 7 hours after the chest pain returned was 22% of the total CPK. The follow-up ECG was consistent with subendocardial myocardial infarction. Surgery was postponed indefinitely, and the patient was transferred to a monitored cardiac unit.

The PA catheter presents the opportunity to do more harm than good. A good deal of concern has been expressed about the benefit of the catheter.[3] A major cause of this concern is the lack of understanding and misinterpretation of data derived from the catheter.[4] It is not sufficient to be skilled in the insertion of a PA catheter. Physicians also must be competent in the interpretation and application of the data derived from the catheter.

## REFERENCES

1. Mangano DT. Perioperative cardiac morbidity. Anesthesiology 72:153, 1990.
2. Crawford ES, Morris GC Jr, Howell JF, et al. Operative risk in patients with previous coronary artery bypass. Ann Thorac Surg 26:215, 1978.
3. Robin ED. Death by pulmonary artery flow-directed catheter: Time for a moratorium? Chest 92:727, 1987.
4. Iberti TJ, Fischer EP, Levibowitz AB, et al. A multicenter study of physicians' knowledge of the pulmonary artery catheter. JAMA 264:2928, 1990.

# CHAPTER 5

# *The Surgical Patient and Renal Failure*

Ricardo Correa-Rotter • Mark E. Rosenberg

## CASE 1

A 70-year-old diabetic man was admitted to the SICU with severe chest pain. An ECG demonstrated characteristic myocardial ischemic changes for which medical treatment was established. The patient's clinical course evolved as unstable angina with poor therapeutic response. Emergency coronary arteriography and ventriculogram were performed (120 ml of nonionic intravenous contrast medium), which revealed severe three-vessel disease. Past medical history was significant for type II diabetes mellitus diagnosed about 18 years earlier, systemic hypertension since age 48, and hypercholesterolemia.

The physical examination revealed a pale, anxious patient. BP was 150/100 mm Hg, pulse 88, and temperature 97.5° F. Mucosal hydration and skin turgor were adequate. The cardiac examination revealed an $S_3$ gallop and no murmurs. The urine output was normal. Laboratory measurements gave the following values: serum Na, 140 mEq/L; K, 4.2 mEq/L; Cl, 101 mEq/L; $CO_2$ content, 20 mEq/L; BUN, 21 mg/100 ml; PCr, 1.8 mg/dl; blood glucose, 183 mg/dl; Hb, 16.2 g/dl; WBC, 6300/mm$^3$; SGOT, 28 U/ml; CPK, 30 U/ml; and 2+ urinary protein by dipstick. Microscopic examination showed the urine to be normal.

Exposure to an intravenous radiocontrast agent constitutes a well-identified risk factor for the development of acute renal failure (ARF) in specific subpopulations. This patient presents the following risk factors known to be associated with radiocontrast nephrotoxicity: advanced age, renal dysfunction secondary to early diabetic nephropathy, and intake of a large dose (120 ml) of contrast medium (nonionic intravenous). Early identification of these risk factors is mandatory in order to implement prophylactic measures aimed at preventing radiocontrast nephrotoxicity.

Diabetes mellitus by itself does not pose an increased risk for the development of radiocontrast-induced ARF. However, the presence of renal insufficiency does increase the risk for nephrotoxicity. The elevated plasma creatinine (PCr) concentration and the presence of urinary protein are consistent with underlying diabetic renal disease. Creatinine clearance (CrCl) can be estimated with the Cockroft and Gault formula, which factors for the patient's age (70 years old), sex (male), and lean body weight (70 kg):

$$\text{CrCl} = (140 - \text{age}) \times \text{Lean body weight}/(\text{PCr} \times 72)$$

In this case, a PCr of 1.8 mg/dl is accompanied by an estimated CrCl of 38 ml/min.

This chapter can be studied in conjunction with *Essentials of Surgical Critical Care,* edited by Jerome H. Abrams and Frank B. Cerra (St. Louis: Quality Medical Publishing, Inc., 1993), Chapters *9,* 30, and 31. Italicized number indicates the main chapter reference.

Volume depletion is another major risk factor for the development of radiocontrast-induced ARF. Therefore adequate assessment of volume status is mandatory. In this patient the medical history and physical examination revealed no apparent volume status alteration. Insertion of a Swan-Ganz catheter for pulmonary capillary wedge pressure (PCWP) measurement and cardiocirculatory monitoring would provide additional information for the continued evaluation and maintenance of circulating blood volume. These measurements are used in conjunction with the physical examination, urine output, and laboratory measurements.

The following protocol can be used to reduce the risk of development of radiocontrast-induced ARF: intravenous administration of 1 L of 5% dextrose in 0.45% normal saline solution with 25 g of mannitol at 150 ml/hr, beginning 2 hours prior to the procedure, followed by continued hydration for up to 24 hours after the procedure. In this patient cardiovascular function and urine output need to be monitored very closely because mannitol may be contraindicated if a low cardiac output is present. If this is the case, a loop diuretic should be used to maintain adequate urine output in conjunction with adequate hydration.

The patient was taken to the operating room for aortocoronary bypass graft surgery. Cardiopulmonary bypass time was 135 minutes. At the end of the surgery, the following relevant clinical and hemodynamic parameters were recorded: pulse, 135; BP, 105/70; urine output, 20 ml/hr; PCWP, 6 mm Hg; cardiac index (CI), 1.8 L $min^{-1}m^{-2}$; and PCr, 2.3. Thirty-six hours after surgery the patient developed fever and cough accompanied by purulent sputum, and a CXR film showed a right upper lobe alveolar pneumonia. Antibiotic treatment, including administration of an aminoglycoside and a third-generation cephalosporin, was initiated. Oliguria persisted, with urine output of 15 ml/hr, and the PCr increased to 3.

During cardiopulmonary bypass surgery, the patient was subjected to considerable renal hypoperfusion. Although the circulatory compromise could not have been avoided in this case, maintenance of an adequate blood flow and perfusion pressure during the procedure and limitation of the cardiopulmonary bypass time to the minimum necessary are measures that are likely to reduce the risk of ARF.

Significant cardiac dysfunction (CI of 1.8) and oliguria were present in the immediate postoperative period. Continued renal circulatory compromise constitutes another risk factor for the development of ARF. The patient's cardiac function should be optimized, and volume status needs to be monitored closely to preserve the fragile fluid balance in this patient. Urinary indexes such as FENa and continued monitoring of urine output and PCr are important parameters to follow in this patient, who has suffered multiple consecutive renal insults.

The recent exposure to intravenous radiocontrast medium in the preoperative period also could be a factor in the renal dysfunction that the patient manifests in the postoperative period since administration of a prophylactic regimen does not eliminate the possibility of development of ARF, particularly in patients with multiple associated risk factors.

The patient developed infectious pneumonia in the postoperative period. This intercurrent medical complication clearly justifies the use of antibiotics. The aminoglycoside prescribed undergoes renal excretion and has potential for nephrotoxicity. Whenever possible, nephrotoxic agents for which adequate antimicrobial alternatives exist should be avoided. In the presence of renal dysfunction, determining the dosage of therapeutic agents must always take into account the patient's age, lean body weight, current glomerular filtration rate, as well as the pharmacokinetics of the drug in order to avoid further renal injury or accumulation of the drug to toxic levels.

## CASE 2

A 42-year-old insulin-dependent diabetic woman was admitted to the emergency room. She complained of nausea, vomiting, and severe right lower quadrant abdominal pain that was exacerbated by motion and cough. Her medical history was significant for insulin-dependent diabetes mellitus diagnosed 23 years earlier. Over the last 12 years she had developed multiple diabetic complications including neuropathy, retinopathy, and nephropathy. At age 34 she was noted to have developed proteinuria (1.3 g/24 hr) and hypertension (BP 150/105), and her PCr was 1.2. Four years before she had had an acute myocardial infarction complicated by congestive heart failure, which responded favorably to medical treatment. At age 40 she developed lower extremity edema and nephrotic range proteinuria (5 g/24 hr), and her PCr was 2.8. The treatment of the patient's renal insufficiency and nephrotic syndrome included dietary restriction of protein, potassium, sodium, and phosphorous, as well as loop diuretics, vasodilators, and oral calcium carbonate.

The physical examination revealed a pale, restless patient. BP was 115/65, pulse 108, temperature 99° F. The chest examination revealed no abnormalities. Right lower quadrant abdominal tenderness was present. Peripheral examination revealed pitting edema to her ankles, absence of sensation in a stocking distribution of both legs, abolished ankle reflexes, and diminished distal pulses in both legs.

Laboratory measurements were Hb, 13 g/dl; WBC, 16,300/mm$^3$; platelets, 354,000/mm$^3$; serum Na, 147 mEq/L; K, 6.7 mEq/L; Cl, 111 mEq/L; $CO_2$ content, 14 mEq/L; BUN, 84 mg/dl; Cr, 5.6 mg/dl; blood glucose, 423 mg/dl; albumin, 2.9 g/dl; Ca, 7.5 mg/dl; serum phosphorus, 5 mg/dl; 4+ urinary protein by dipstick, and abundant granular casts in the microscopic examination of the urine. Plain abdominal x-ray examination gave normal results. A clinical diagnosis of acute appendicitis was established, and the patient was evaluated for emergency surgery.

This patient faces an acute abdominal condition requiring emergency surgical intervention. Of major significance in the preoperative evaluation are her renal insufficiency and volume status since she has nephrotic syndrome and advanced renal failure due to diabetic nephropathy. Careful assessment of her actual cardiovascular condition is also mandatory because she had a myocardial infarction at age 38 that was accompanied by an episode of congestive heart failure.

In spite of the presence of moderate lower extremity edema, the patient has clinical and laboratory evidence of intravascular volume depletion probably secondary to vomiting (tachycardia, BP of 115/65 in a previously known hypertensive patient, hypernatremia, and a Hb of 13, which is probably inappropriately high for the degree of renal failure). Fluid administration in this patient is not without risk because overhydration and pulmonary edema may ensue. Therefore the insertion of a Swan-Ganz catheter for cardiocirculatory monitoring is clearly indicated to evaluate her volume status and safely replace intravascular fluid losses. Hyperglycemia is an important contributor to her fluid and electrolyte imbalance and should be promptly treated.

Hyperkalemia (6.7 mEq/L in this case) may be a life-threatening condition because it favors the development of cardiac dysrhythmias. Anesthesia poses an added risk for hyperkalemia-related dysrhythmias because the muscle relaxant succinylcoline may increase serum potassium by an additional 0.5 mEq/L. In evaluating hyperkalemia, it is useful to estimate its severity by considering both serum potassium levels and the ECG. Insulin treatment, indicated in this case for the management of severe hyperglycemia, will lower serum potassium by effecting an internal redistribution (shift of potassium to the intracellular space). Oral administration of a cationic-exchange resin such as sodium polystyrene sulfonate (e.g., Kayexelate), intended to remove potassium from the body, would be contraindicated in this case because of the nature of the surgical emergency. Careful evaluation of the patient's acid-base status should be performed, including ABG analysis, before a decision about specific therapeutic measures is made.

Of relevance is the PCr of 5.6 mg/dl, which in this case corresponds to an estimated CrCl of 14 ml/min (42 years old and lean body weight of 55 kg). This is probably related to a prerenal exacerbation of the patient's diabetic nephropathy. The dosages of drugs excreted by the kidney need to be appropriately adjusted.

Since bleeding disorders are common in the uremic patient because of platelet dysfunction and anemia, bleeding time should be determined; if it is elevated, treatment should be provided to restore hemostasis prior to surgery.

A Swan-Ganz pulmonary catheter was placed, and the following relevant data were obtained: pulse, 112; BP, 120/75; PCWP, 2 mm Hg; CI , 2.7 $L/min^{-1} \cdot m^{-2}$; and systemic vascular resistance, 1300 $dyne/sec/cm^5$. Urine output during the first hour after admission was 20 ml.

The following laboratory results were obtained. ABG analysis: pH, 7.35; partial pressure of carbon dioxide, 37 mm Hg; partial pressure of oxygen, 88 mm Hg; plasma $HCO_3^-$, 15 mEq/L. Bleeding time was 15 minutes (normal 1 to 4 minutes by Duke method). The ECG showed moderate T-wave peaking.

For intravascular volume replacement, normal saline solution should be started at 150 ml/hr. When the blood glucose falls to <250 mg/dl, 5% glucose in normal saline solution should be started. The volume of fluids infused is determined by monitoring PCWP and urine output. Blood pH and bicarbonate determinations show a state of compensated metabolic acidosis, yet intravenous bicarbonate administration (initially 50 mEq of $NaHCO_3$) would be indicated because it will favor potassium shift to the intracellular space, improve the acid-base state, and contribute to the management of volume depletion. ABGs should be carefully monitored because administration of excess $HCO_3^-$ can lead to rapid alkalinization with detrimental effects on oxygen delivery to tissues. Improvement of the uremic bleeding tendency may be obtained by administering 1-deamino-8-arginine vasopressin (DDAVP) (0.3 μg/kg in 50 ml of isotonic saline solution over 30 minutes). A beneficial effect is seen within 1 hour after its administration and lasts for several hours. Tolerance may develop with repeated doses.

The patient received 1 L of normal saline solution, a continuous infusion of insulin, 50 mEq of $NaHCO_3$, and 16 μg of DDAVP. The patient's PCWP increased to 8 mm Hg, and urine output increased to 50 ml/hr. Repeat laboratory results were as follows: serum Na, 145 mEq/L; K, 4.8 mEq/L; Cl, 104 mEq/L; $CO_2$ content, 18; BUN, 80 mg/dl; Cr, 5.4; glucose, 200 mg/dl.

The patient was taken to the operating room where an inflamed appendix was removed without complication. Urine output during surgery was 70 ml/hr. Postoperatively the patient was transferred to the SICU.

This case emphasized the importance of careful preoperative assessment and management of the renal patient who requires emergency surgery.

# CHAPTER 6

# *Airway Management*

Ian J. Gilmour

## CASE 1

A 63-year-old woman was admitted to the SICU approximately 3 days following an emergency colectomy for a ruptured diverticulum. Her history was significant only for mild osteoarthritis. She was otherwise healthy. Her postoperative course was characterized by spiking temperatures and an increasing WBC count. On postoperative day 3, she became progressively more dyspneic and required transfer to the SICU for intubation and mechanical ventilation with high levels of positive end-expiratory pressure and a fraction of inspired oxygen of 0.6. A tentative diagnosis of adult respiratory distress syndrome was made. On the evening of the patient's admission to the SICU, a nurse noted that the volume alarm of the patient's ventilator was sounding repeatedly. After auscultation over the trachea, the respiratory therapist reported a cuff leak. The leak was eliminated by the addition of 3 cc of air to the endotracheal tube cuff. Approximately 3 hours later, the situation recurred. More air was added to the cuff, and the tube to the pilot balloon was clamped. ABG measurements obtained at this time showed some deterioration compared to those obtained earlier in the day.

- *What should you do next?*

This patient's condition deteriorated because a cuff leak prevented positive end-expiratory pressure (PEEP) from achieving its full efficacy; there also may have been a decrease in minute ventilation. The differential diagnosis includes cuff failure and partial extubation; partial extubation is more likely. To establish the diagnosis, several options are available. A simple first step is to estimate the depth of the endotracheal tube (ETT). In an adult woman the tube should be at 20 to 21 cm at the teeth; in a man, 22 to 23 cm. In many SICUs it is routine to note the depth of the tube at initial intubation. With this information, diagnosis of outward migration of the tube should be easier. A CXR film also can be used to locate the tip of the ETT. Another alternative is palpation of the trachea while injecting 2 to 3 cc of air into the pilot balloon. This procedure can be helpful in localizing the cuff but should be used with care in an awake patient.

A repeat ABG analysis showed pH as 7.35; arterial partial pressure of carbon dioxide ($Pa_{CO_2}$), 45; arterial partial pressure of oxygen ($Pa_{O_2}$), 61; fraction of inspired oxygen ($F_{IO_2}$), 0.6; and PEEP, 15 cm $H_2O$. $F_{IO_2}$ was increased to 1. The CXR film obtained after initial intubation was unavailable, and there would be a delay in obtaining a new one. The depth of the tube at the time of intubation had not been recorded. On examination of the patient, it was found

This chapter can be studied in conjunction with *Essentials of Surgical Critical Care*, edited by Jerome H. Abrams and Frank B. Cerra (St. Louis: Quality Medical Publishing, Inc., 1993), Chapter 11.

that the 19-cm mark on the ETT was at the patient's teeth, and the adhesive tape around the ETT had slipped. Palpation of the ETT cuff confirmed that the cuff was above the hyoid. The anesthesiologist was called to reintubate the patient.

Manipulation of the airway in a patient with severe respiratory dysfunction can be extremely hazardous. Assuming that the diagnosis of adult respiratory distress syndrome (ARDS) is correct, one can predict that this patient's lung compliance will be markedly diminished. Two problems arise. First, mask ventilation will be inefficient; there is a high probability of ventilating the stomach and promoting regurgitation and aspiration. Second, as functional residual capacity is reduced, the patient will desaturate very rapidly during the reintubation attempt. For these reasons, patient safety would be improved if there were an alterative to reintubation.

The anesthesiologist reintubated the patient by advancing the existing ETT over a stylet. The patient was monitored with a pulse oximeter throughout the procedure. The stylet was marked at a point 10 cm longer than the ETT. After the patient was sedated and the stylet was lubricated, the patient was disconnected from the ventilator. The stylet was introduced quickly but gently into the ETT. It passed easily to the mark previously mentioned. The cuff was deflated and the tube advanced to the 22 cm mark at the teeth. The patient coughed. The cuff was reinflated and the patient was reconnected to the ventilator. By cuff palpation, the tube position was acceptable. Arterial oxygen saturation ($Spo_2$) reached a nadir of 87% during the procedure but was soon back to 96%. Partial pressure of end-tidal carbon dioxide ($Petco_2$) was noted to be 28 mm Hg. A CXR film subsequently confirmed that the tube was positioned appropriately. Results from an ABG analysis obtained one half hour later were pH, 7.45; $Paco_2$, 35; and $Pao_2$, 95.

Under these circumstances, the volume of air in the ETT cuff can be enormous. In this case 23 cc of air was removed. Accordingly, a large (30 cc) syringe should be available for this purpose. Attempts to advance an ETT without a stylet will almost always fail in orally intubated patients because after several hours in a patient, the tube is so soft and malleable that when advanced, it is likely to kink rather than progress. This kinking often completely displaces the tube tip from the glottis. In nasally intubated patients, advancing the tube blindly is more often successful, which is fortunate because changing the tube over a stylet is not an option in nasally intubated patients. Whatever method is chosen, the ETT cuff must be deflated completely before an attempt is made to advance the tube. The following equipment should be available as a backup: (1) bag/valve/mask, (2) oxygen and suction sources, (3) a functioning laryngoscope, (4) a selection of endotracheal tubes, (5) muscle relaxant and sedative or anesthetics, and (6) tracheostomy and cricothyrotomy trays.

## CASE 2

The patient was a morbidly obese (142 kg) 42-year-old woman. She had undergone a total abdominal hysterectomy for cervical cancer and was found early in the morning of the first postoperative day unresponsive and apneic with vomitus on the pillow beside her. Basic life support was initiated. Ventilation was attempted initially with bag/valve/mask but was unsatisfactory. The physician on call attempted to intubate the patient orally several times without success. Upon his arrival with the rest of the code team, the anesthesiologist also attempted to visualize the larynx but was unable to do so. After suctioning the airway, he was able to begin ventilation with bag/valve/mask. Heart rhythm improved from sinus bradycardia to sinus tachycardia following several doses of epinephrine. BP stabilized to 160/90. $Spo_2$ was 93% with an $Fio_2$ of 1.

- *What should be done now?*

With ample evidence of regurgitation and aspiration of gastric contents, it would appear to be necessary to establish an airway for ongoing mechanical ventilatory support in this patient. With the patient ventilated adequately by bag/valve/mask, some time is available to assess the options. A possibility is a modified Seldinger approach to oral intubation using a guidewire threaded through the cricothyroid membrane and back through the mouth. Further efforts at direct laryngoscopy are not likely to be successful after many failed attempts. Edema and hemorrhage from multiple previous laryngoscopies also will make fiberoptic laryngoscopy and blind nasal intubation difficult. Surgical approaches (cricothyrotomy, tracheostomy) are viable options.

While vital signs remained stable, ventilation with bag/valve/mask was insufficient to elevate the $Spo_2$ above 93% even with an $Fio_2$ of 1. The anesthesiologist decided to perform an oral intubation over a guidewire passed retrograde through the cricothyroid membrane. This was accomplished without difficulty using a 6 mm ETT, and the patient was transferred to the SICU.

Over the next 48 hours, the patient's respiratory status continued to deteriorate, and progressive increases in ventilatory support were required. Fortunately, the patient's neurologic status improved dramatically. She began to complain of severe pain in the region of her larynx. Upon fiberoptic laryngoscopy, the otolaryngology consultants observed marked edema and inflammation of the glottis, some mucosal ulcerations, and what appeared to be dislocation of the left arytenoid cartilage. Because the ETT in place was rather small (6 mm ID), it was decided that a tracheostomy would be performed at the same time as relocation of the arytenoid cartilage. This procedure was uneventful; the tracheostomy tube used was short. The patient's general condition continued to improve, but about 36 hours after tracheostomy, while turning the patient, the nurse heard the pressure alarm on the ventilator, and the patient's $Spo_2$ began to deteriorate rapidly. The ventilator was disconnected, and the nurse attempted bag/valve ventilation and called for help.

- *What are your options?*

The choice of a short tracheostomy tube in this patient was unfortunate because the tube is rather too short for a morbidly obese patient. Movement of the patient or ventilator circuit is likely to cause the tube tip to slip outside the trachea. Attempts at ventilation through the tracheostomy tube should be abandoned until it can be confirmed that the tube is correctly placed. Ventilation through a malpositioned tube will result in emphysema of surrounding tissue with compression of the upper airway and the risk of pneumothorax and pneumomediastinum. One should attempt to initiate ventilation by bag/valve/mask and call for anesthesia to attempt oral intubation and for help skilled enough to recannulate the stoma of a fresh tracheostomy. A selection of tracheostomy tubes should be available along with a tracheostomy set containing appropriate instruments. An adequate source of light is also necessary.

The tracheostomy tube was removed, and bag/valve/mask ventilation was begun with an assistant plugging the patient's tracheostomy stoma during inspiration. The anesthesiologist arrived and after administration of succinyl dicholine and atropine was able to intubate the patient translaryngeally. The tube was advanced so that the cuff was distal to the stoma. The airway was suctioned and manual ventilation was continued. After accomplishing hemostasis at the stomal site, the senior surgery resident used tracheostomy instruments to visualize the tracheal stoma. The ETT was slowly withdrawn, and a suction catheter was introduced into the stoma. With the catheter used as a guide, the stoma was recannulated with an 8 mm ID Portex (Concora Portex, Keene, N.H.) extended-length tracheostomy tube. The suction catheter was withdrawn. Correct placement was confirmed with capnometry and auscultation. Mechanical ventilation was resumed. The patient was discharged from the SICU 9 days after the tracheostomy.

Pitfalls in airway management in patients whose tracheostomy is advertently decannulated include the following:

1. Continued attempts to ventilate through the displaced tracheostomy tube. Only if a suction catheter can be passed easily through the tube and capnometry confirms correct placement should ventilation through the tracheostomy tube be reinstituted.
2. Repeated efforts to recannulate without proper lighting and equipment. Although occasionally recannulation can be successful (e.g., using a suction catheter as a guide), most commonly the result is more bleeding and trauma. Ventilation should be attempted, as it was in this case, by bag/valve/mask and/or translaryngeal intubation.
3. Failure to attempt endotracheal intubation because it was previously unsuccessful. In this case, edema was much diminished because the airway trauma had occurred almost 96 hours before. Even in patients with epiglottitis, who often are admitted with almost complete airway obstruction, oral intubation should be attempted.
4. Failure to use the consistent presence of carbon dioxide in expired gas as the indicator for appropriate placement. Dependence on breath sounds in particular is fraught with hazard in these patients.
5. Failure to correct the primary problem by replacing the initial tracheostomy tube with one more appropriate to the patient's anatomy. This failure almost guarantees that the problem will recur.

# CHAPTER 7

# *Pulmonary Embolism*

Mark D. Cipolle

## CASE 1

A 59-year-old man underwent a low anterior resection for adenocarcinoma of the rectum. His medical history was significant for the smoking of two packs of cigarettes daily. The operation was done in the lithotomy position and was uncomplicated. When the patient arrived at the general care service after surgery, pneumatic compression boots and elastic stockings were placed on both lower extremities. For the first several hours postoperatively, the patient's course was uneventful. During the night, the house officer was called to evaluate the patient's agitation and inability to sleep. Morphine sulfate and diazepam were ordered. At 4 AM the patient was quite dyspneic, BP was 70/40 mm Hg, and pulse was 140 beats/min. Fluids were administered, and the patient was rushed to the SICU.

On arrival at the SICU, the patient's BP was 80/50 mm Hg, and the respiratory rate was 50. With the patient breathing 50% oxygen by mask, an ABG analysis showed a pH of 7.45, partial pressure of carbon dioxide ($Paco_2$) of 30 mm Hg, and partial pressure of oxygen ($Pao_2$) of 45 mm Hg. The patient was intubated, intravenous fluids were continued, and a pulmonary artery (PA) catheter was inserted. Cardiac index (CI) was 2.1 L/min, PA pressures were 65/50, and the pulmonary capillary wedge pressure (PCWP) was 8 mm Hg. The central venous pressure (CVP) was 18 cm $H_2O$. An ECG showed a right bundle branch block, right ventricular strain pattern, and nonspecific ST-T segment changes. The Hb was 11.5 g/dl (0.5 g/dl less than preoperatively), and electrolyte concentrations were normal. Lactate concentration was 3.1 mmol. Fluid administration was continued. The CVP increased to 24 cm $H_2O$, but the PCWP increased to 10 mm Hg. The systolic BP remained below 85.

Since the Hb was not significantly changed and no significant ST-segment changes were seen on the ECG, hemorrhage or acute myocardial infarction is not a likely mechanism for the patient's decompensation. In consultation with the surgeon, the decision is made to heparinize the patient with a bolus of 10,000 U, and a constant infusion is started at 1500 U/hr. Several findings suggest pulmonary embolism (PE) as the correct diagnosis: agitation, hypoxemia, hypotension, elevated PA pressures, elevated CVP, decreased PCWP, and a right strain pattern on the ECG. The patient is in a high-risk category for the development of perioperative deep venous thrombosis (DVT). Risk factors include age, malignancy, and type of surgical procedure. Pelvic surgery and the lithotomy position are higher risk than supine abdominal laparotomy procedures. Of note is the timing of DVT prophylaxis. Although the surgeon had good intentions

This chapter can be studied in conjunction with *Essentials of Surgical Critical Care,* edited by Jerome H. Abrams and Frank B. Cerra (St. Louis: Quality Medical Publishing, Inc., 1993), Chapter 12.

in ordering compression boots, they should be in place before the patient is positioned on the operating table. The patient is at highest risk to develop DVT *during* surgery.

To confirm the diagnosis of DVT and PE, one should first decide whether the patient is a candidate for thrombolytic therapy. Although this patient had surgery fewer than 18 hours ago, he had an anterior resection performed with no untoward events. The possibility of mortality from this suspected "massive" PE seems to substantially outweigh a significant bleeding risk during lytic therapy. This patient should have pulmonary angiography performed without delay to confirm the presence or absence of a PE and to obtain a baseline assessment of the extent of clot before starting lytic therapy. With the high index of suspicion and the instability of the patient, precious time is consumed in obtaining Doppler ultrasound studies of the lower extremities. A ventilation/perfusion (V/Q) scan may not be necessary in this clinical setting.

> The pulmonary arteriogram then showed a saddle PE. Urokinase was started via the same femoral vein approach used for the pulmonary arteriogram.

With the current protocol being followed, a loading dose of urokinase followed by a constant infusion is initiated. The patient also should be maintained on heparin during urokinase infusion to keep the partial thromboplastin time about two times control. Fibrinogen concentrations also should be monitored, and the urokinase rate should be adjusted if the concentration drops below 0.2 mg/dl.

> The patient improved dramatically in just a few hours. Hypoxemia, cardiac output, PA pressures, and arterial BP returned to normal limits. Radiographically, the PE was nearly totally resolved in 6 hours.

Other therapeutic options should be ready in case lytic therapy fails or the patient sustains clinically significant bleeding. In either of these events, pulmonary embolectomy would need to be considered. This patient should be maintained on heparin therapy and then converted to coumadin therapy for 3 months.

## CASE 2

> A 42-year-old woman became dyspneic. Concomitantly, oxygen saturation, as measured by a pulse oximeter, decreased from 97% to 85% on 2 L of oxygen. The patient had had an uneventful cholecystectomy performed on the previous day and had just received parenteral meperidine for pain. She was mildly obese and healthy. Postoperatively, she received subcutaneous heparin 5000 U q 12 hr, but no heparin was administered preoperatively. Her temperature was 101.4° F; respiratory rate, 30; pulse, 104 beats/min; and BP, 120/80 mm Hg. The physical examination was unremarkable except for diminished breath sounds in both lung bases with some scattered ronchi. CXR film, ECG, electrolytes, and CBC results all were normal. ABG analysis on 2 L of oxygen revealed pH of 7.33, $Paco_2$ of 30 mm Hg, and $Pao_2$ of 55 mm Hg.

This patient should be evaluated for DVT and PE. Her risk was moderate, and her perioperative DVT prophylaxis was inadequate. The physician should obtain duplex Doppler ultrasound studies of her lower extremities and a V/Q scan.

> In this case the duplex ultrasound studies showed no evidence of DVT in either of the lower extremities, and the V/Q scan was indeterminate.

With this information, one should obtain sequential duplex Doppler ultrasound studies of the patient's lower extremities to ensure that clots do not appear at the level of the knee or above. Hull et al.[1] recommend six studies over 2 weeks. This patient does not need to be anticoagulated. One might argue that negative duplex studies would negate the need for a V/Q scan. Hull et al.[2] showed that as many as 30% of patients with negative results on impedance plethysmography for lower extremity DVT had positive pulmonary arteriograms. These findings support the practice of not obtaining a V/Q scan only in those patients with a very low suspicion of PE or a clearly identified other cause for their pulmonary problems. In this case the patient's desaturation was probably caused by postoperative atelectasis and, perhaps, oversedation. Nonetheless, she deserved an evaluation to rule out DVT and PE.

## CASE 3

A 17-year-old woman was involved in a roll-over motor vehicle crash and was ejected 45 feet from the car out the back window. She was found unconscious at the scene with low BP, bleeding from the scalp, a right flail chest, and bilateral lower extremity deformities. The patient was intubated, an IV line was started, and she was rushed to a trauma unit. Administration of fluids and blood and placement of a right chest tube stabilized the BP. Evaluation revealed diffuse cerebral swelling, a right flail chest with hemopneumothorax, pulmonary contusion, fractures of the pelvic ramus and right acetabulum, a right subtrochanteric femoral fracture, and a left open tibiofibular fracture with degloving. The results of peritoneal lavage were negative. An intracranial pressure monitor, placed while the patient's open tibiofibular fracture was debrided, read 30 mm Hg. Before leaving the operating room, the orthopedic surgeon placed a pin in the patient's right leg for femur traction.

- *What is DVT prophylaxis for this patient?*

The patient cannot have anticoagulants because of her closed head injury. Neither of her lower extremities is available for compression boots. Some institutions would place a prophylactic vena caval filter in this patient. Alternatively, no prophylaxis could be used and the patient's lower extremities could be monitored for the development of clots through bedside duplex venography. Another possibility is placement of sequential compression devices on both upper extremities as DVT prophylaxis. Several references have shown that these devices have a systemic lytic effect when placed on the legs.[3-5] In addition, it has been shown that there is quantitatively more fibrinolytic activity in arm veins compared to leg veins.[6] Most important, Knight and Dawson[7] showed that intermittent compression of the arms during and after surgery reduced the incidence of DVT in the legs by 50% and maintained blood fibrinolytic activity at preoperative values.

### REFERENCES


1. Hull RD, Raskob GE, Coules G, et al. A new non-invasive management strategy for patients with suspected pulmonary embolism. Arch Intern Med 149:2549, 1989.
2. Hull RD, Hirsch J, Carter CJ, et al. Pulmonary angiography, ventilation scanning, and venography for clinically suspected pulmonary embolism with abnormal perfusion lung scan. Ann Intern Med 98:891, 1983.
3. Allenby F, Pflug JJ, Boardman L, Calvin JS. Effects of external pneumatic compression on fibrinolysis in men. Lancet 2:1412, 1973.
4. Tarnaz TJ, Rohr PA, Davidson AG, et al. Pneumatic calf compression, fibrinolysis, and the prevention of deep venous thrombosis. Surgery 88:489, 1980.

5. Inada K, Koike S, Shirai N, et al. Effects of intermittent pneumatic leg compression for prevention of postoperative deep venous thrombosis with special reference to fibrinolytic activity. Am J Surg 155:602, 1988.
6. Pandolfi M, Robertson B, Isaacsson S, Nilsson IM. Fibrinolytic activity of human veins in arms and legs. Thromb Diath Hemorrh 20:247, 1968.
7. Knight MTM, Dawson R. Effect of intermittent compression of the arms on deep venous thrombosis in the legs. Lancet 2:1265, 1976.

## SUGGESTED READING

Goldhaber SZ. Recent advances in the diagnosis and lytic therapy of pulmonary embolism. Chest 99:1735, 1991.

# CHAPTER 8

## *Nursing Considerations*

**Becky Jo Lekander • Beth M. Nelson**

### CASE

A previously healthy 31-year-old woman was admitted to the SICU with hemorrhagic and necrotizing pancreatitis of unknown etiology. The patient was hypotensive on admission from another hospital. A CT scan showed an edematous pancreas with fatty liver infiltration, a distended gallbladder, and ductal dilation. Urine output at the time of admission was approximately 20 ml/hr; the patient was being volume resuscitated. A diagnosis of gallstone pancreatitis was made.

Respiratory distress increased, and the patient was intubated on the second hospital day. Her temperature rose to 103.1° F. The lactate concentration was 2.6 mmol. Antibiotic therapy was initiated.

Three days later the patient remained febrile. She maintained a persistent hypermetabolic/septic state, with decreased systemic vascular resistance and a high cardiac output and cardiac index.

Nursing care focused on providing volume resuscitation, supporting ventilation, suctioning secretions, and maintaining circulatory support with vasoactive medications. Of primary concern to the nurses was diagnosing the presence or absence of patient and family coping skills. Consistent nursing care by a team of three to four registered nurses provided a coordinated plan of nursing care, which was communicated to the entire health team. The nurses provided an essential communication link between the family and the multitude of consulting physicians and health team members.

The patient required inotropic medications and ventilatory support. Results from cultures were negative. Because of worsening hypermetabolism, continued fever, and hemodynamic instability, pancreatic abscess vs. pancreatic necrosis was suspected. At laparotomy, severe hemorrhagic pancreatitis with large areas of necrosis was found.

During the following 2 weeks the patient was returned to the operating room many times for multiple debridements of pancreatic and necrotic retroperitoneal tissue. The contaminated abdominal wound remained opened and packed.

In the postoperative period the patient required large volumes of blood products. Her open wound required wet-to-dry soaks three times per day with triple antibiotic and amphotericin

This chapter can be studied in conjunction with *Essentials of Surgical Critical Care,* edited by Jerome H. Abrams and Frank B. Cerra (St. Louis: Quality Medical Publishing, Inc., 1993), Chapter 13.

B solutions. Because of the patient's large wound and the loss of surrounding vascular integrity, the dressing changes required extra time. Collaboration between physicians and nurses allowed joint assessments and evaluation of wound healing. Physicians and nurses used the decision tree shown in Fig. 8-1 to determine the appropriate type of therapeutic bed. After consideration, an air-fluidized bed was selected.

> The patient continued to receive antimicrobial drugs. Her fever disappeared, and she was weaned from inotropic support.

Despite the need for frequent dressing changes and mechanical ventilation, the patient was gradually mobilized. She progressed from using a mechanical lift to get out of bed to eventually

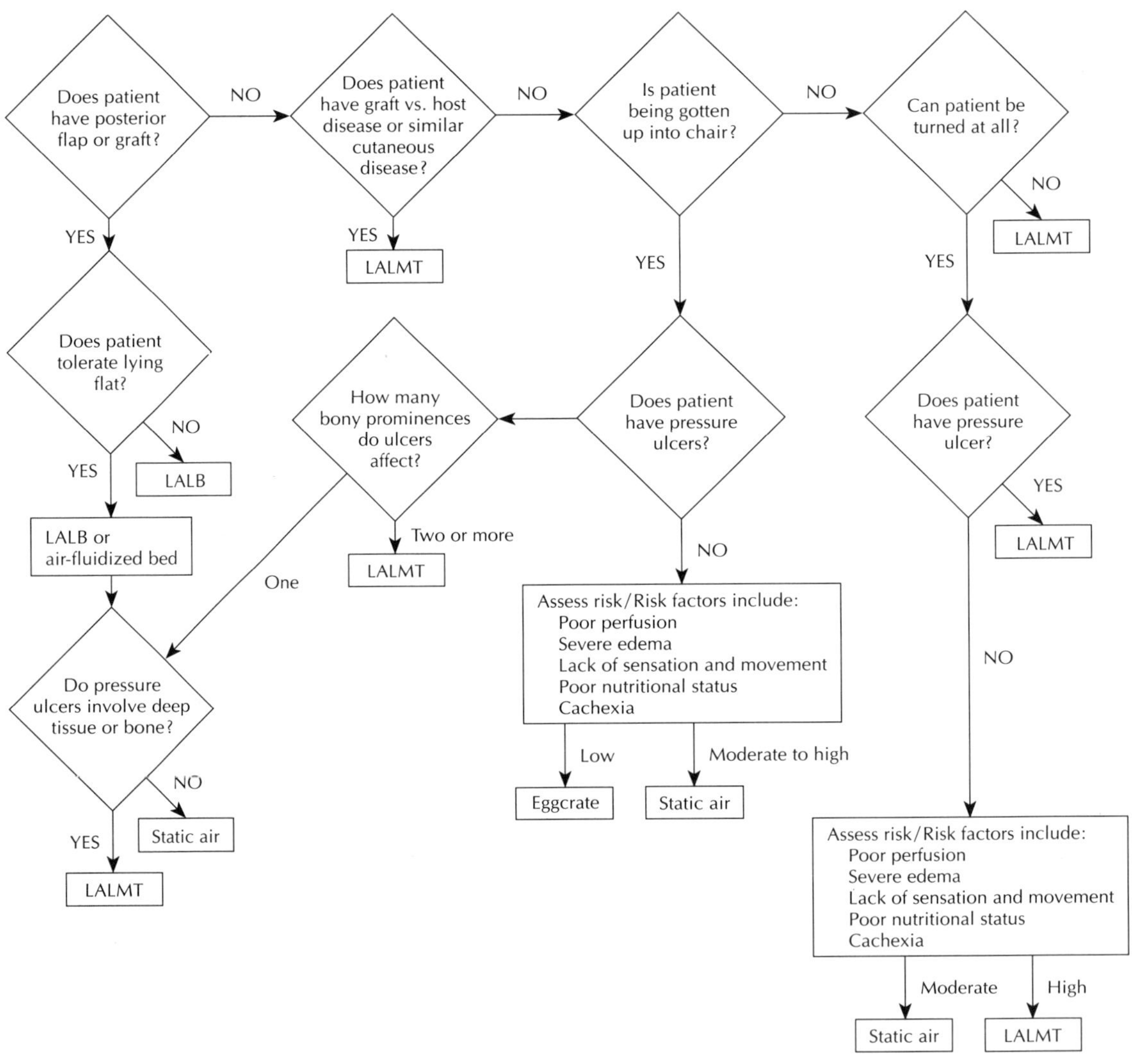


**FIG 8-1** Decision tree for use of pressure-reducing products in management of patients with complicated wounds or complications of immobility. LALT, low-air-loss topper; LALB, low-air-loss bed. *Note:* Chart does not include RotoRest bed for spinal stabilization or Burke Obese bed for large patients. (Courtesy Kathryn Hoyman, R.N., Minneapolis.)

bearing her weight to transfer herself to a chair. The nurses were careful to position the patient in full Fowler's position while in the chair. This position increases tidal volume, helps to mobilize secretions, and minimizes fluid shift. Initially, moving the patient from bed to chair required the help of many staff members. Eventually the patient progressed to using a walker with minimal assistance.

> The patient was intubated and ventilated for 1 month. A tracheostomy was then performed, and the tube remained in place for 2 months. The patient was weaned via a combination pressure support–CPAP mask (BIPAP) intermittently with continuous positive airway pressure.

Weaning the patient from mechanical ventilatory support was a collaborative effort among the patient, respiratory therapists, nurses, and physicians. Nurses provided consistent information and appropriate reassurance to the patient and family during the weaning process. The patient was eventually weaned from mechanical ventilation and inotropic support, and she was transferred to general care. Dressing changes and rehabilitation were continued for the remainder of her hospital course. The patient was discharged, and her family continued to provide dressing changes twice a day.

This patient also required ongoing teaching regarding nutrition, dressing changes, activity, and exercise.

The nursing staff communicated with the family regularly throughout the patient's hospital course. The nurse became the coordinator of the patient's care. Of major interest to the health team were dressing changes to the open abdominal wound, encouraging the patient to recognize the goals achieved during hospitalization, dealing with her attention-seeking and demanding behavior, setting limits, and providing consistent nursing care.

# CHAPTER 9

## *Role of Rehabilitation*

Elizabeth A. Davis

### CASE 1

A 24-year-old man fell 20 feet while working at a construction site. He landed on his left shoulder and rib cage and struck the back of his head. The man noticed acute onset of numbness in his arms and legs and was unable to move his extremities. X-ray films revealed facet fractures of C6 and C7 vertebrae with subluxation, rib fractures, and a left scapula fracture. Physical examination revealed motor function to C7 and sensation to C8. The patient also had a neurogenic bladder and bowel. He was placed in Gardner-Wells tongs for initial spinal stabilization.

- *What are your initial rehabilitation objectives?*

Preservation of joint mobility and remaining muscle strength are the initial objectives. Of importance is the fact that the extent of the spinal injury may not be known for several weeks. Development of fixed joint contractures may prevent the patient from having functional motor recovery even if the neurologic injury resolves. Appropriate bed positioning and use of splints should be ordered.

The patient should receive physical therapy for range of motion and strengthening exercises. Occupational therapy should be done for evaluation of the patient's upper extremity function. Adaptive equipment can be provided early in treatment so that the patient can maintain some functional independence.

The patient's muscle tone should be monitored, and antispasticity medications, such as baclofen, should be used as necessary. The patient should be lying on a pressure relief mattress to prevent skin breakdown.

An intermittent bladder catheterization program should be initiated. A neurogenic bowel program should be started to prevent obstipation if no ileus is present.

One week after admission, the patient began moving his left leg, quadriceps, and gastrocnemius.

- *What is your clinical impression? What is your plan?*

The spinal injury is incomplete, a situation that provides hope for further neurologic recovery. The returning muscle function should be strengthened by active exercise or functional electrical stimulation.

---

This chapter can be studied in conjunction with *Essentials of Surgical Critical Care,* edited by Jerome H. Abrams and Frank B. Cerra (St. Louis: Quality Medical Publishing, Inc., 1993), Chapter 14.

The patient should be gotten out of bed as soon as possible after spinal stabilization. Early rehabilitation intervention and transfer to a spinal cord rehabilitation unit have been shown to improve final outcome and decrease complications.

## CASE 2

A 16-year-old man was admitted to the emergency department after his bicycle was struck by a car. His initial Glasgow Coma Scale score was 7. He would not open his eyes. The patient moved his left side spontaneously but had decreased movement of his right side. His right arm exhibited flexor tone. His right leg exhibited extensor tone. The patient made no sounds and followed no commands. Initial CT scan showed diffuse edema with an intracerebral hemorrhage in the left temporal lobe. No surgical intervention was indicated.

- *What rehabilitation intervention is indicated?*

Early rehabilitation, an important component of patient management, is directed toward maintaining range of motion of all joints. After the patient's medical condition has been stabilized, musculoskeletal complications can prolong hospitalization and decrease the final level of independence achieved.

Passive range of motion should be performed to all extremities. Special attention should be directed to the increased tone in the right arm and leg. A right handsplint should be fabricated by an occupational therapist to inhibit the flexor tone.

The splint should be worn for 2 hours and then taken off for 2 hours to prevent skin breakdown. The skin should be checked for any pressure areas. If necessary, the splint should be modified.

A prefabricated or customized foot-drop splint should be applied to the right foot to inhibit the extensor tone. An inhibitory cast can be applied if the splint cannot maintain the range of motion. The cast should be changed every 2 to 3 days to accommodate any increased range of motion obtained.

As the patient's level of consciousness improves, attention should be directed to the patient's communication and cognitive status. Early recognition of deficits facilitates communication among the patient, the medical team, and the patient's family. As soon as the patient's medical condition allows, he should be sitting up in a chair and performing more functional exercise activities.

# SECTION 2 *Guidelines for Pharmacologic Problem-Solving*

## CHAPTER 10

# *Optimization of Drug Doses*

Pamela K. Borchardt-Phelps • Bruce C. Lohr

### CASE 1

A 64-year-old woman weighing 60 kg was being treated in the SICU for postoperative atrial fibrillation. She received 1 mg of intravenous digoxin over 6 hours, which brought her ventricular rate under control. However, atrial fibrillation was still present, and chemical conversion with intravenous procainamide was to be attempted.

- *Calculate an appropriate loading dose of intravenous procainamide for this patient. Assume normal renal function for her age. The desired plasma concentration is 7 mg/L (normal, 4 to 10 mg/L).*

Equation 1 can be used to calculate a loading dose.

EQUATION 1

$$\text{Loading dose} = \frac{(\text{Vd})\,(\text{Cp})}{(\text{S})\,(\text{F})}$$

where

Vd = Volume of distribution
Cp = Desired plasma concentration
S = Fraction of drug that is active moiety
F = Bioavailability

Average pharmacokinetic parameters for procainamide can be obtained from the literature for making initial estimates. Procainamide has a Vd of approximately 2 L/kg, and S is 0.82. Bioavailability for intravenous injections is 1.

$$\text{Loading dose} = \frac{(2\text{ L/kg})\,(60\text{ kg})\,(7\text{ mg/L})}{(0.82)\,(1)}$$

$$\text{Loading dose} = 1024\text{ mg}$$

This chapter can be studied in conjunction with *Essentials of Surgical Critical Care,* edited by Jerome H. Abrams and Frank B. Cerra (St. Louis: Quality Medical Publishing, Inc., 1993), Chapter 15.

This dose would be rounded to 1 g since the drug is manufactured in 1 g vials. The dose should be administered at a rate no faster than 20 mg/min to avoid drug-induced hypotension.

> Several minutes after the loading infusion was completed, the patient's heart rate reverted to sinus rhythm. The patient was to be maintained on continuous intravenous infusion.
>
> - *Calculate an infusion rate that will produce a plasma concentration of 7 mg/L at steady state.*

Equation 2 can be used for this calculation.

EQUATION 2

$$\text{Maintenance dose} = \frac{(\text{Cl})\,(\text{Cp})\,(\tau)}{(\text{S})\,(\text{F})}$$

where

Cl = Clearance
Cp = Desired plasma concentration
$\tau$ = Dosing interval
S = Fraction of drug that is active moiety
F = Bioavailability

The average clearance for procainamide reported in the literature for patients over 60 years of age is 4.3 ml/kg/min, which is 0.26 L/min for this patient.

$$\text{Maintenance dose} = \frac{(0.26\ \text{L/min})\,(7\ \text{mg/L})\,(1\ \text{min})}{(0.82)\,(1)}$$

$$\text{Maintenance dose} = 2.2\ \text{mg/min}$$

This result would be rounded to 2 mg/min for ease of administration.

> A steady-state procainamide plasma concentration of 10 mg/L was obtained 21 hours after the infusion was started. It was decided to reduce the infusion rate to bring the concentration down to 7 mg/L.
>
> - *Calculate the patient's actual procainamide clearance.*

Equation 3 (a rearrangement of Equation 2) can be used for this determination.

EQUATION 3

$$\text{Clearance} = \frac{(\text{S})\,(\text{F})\,(\text{Infusion rate})}{\text{Cp}}$$

$$\text{Clearance} = \frac{(0.82)\,(1)\,(2\ \text{mg/min})}{10\ \text{mg/L}}$$

$$\text{Clearance} = 0.16\ \text{L/min}$$

> - *Calculate a new intravenous infusion rate that will produce a steady-state plasma concentration of 7 mg/L for this patient.*

Equation 2 can be used again, with the patient's actual clearance used instead of a value from the literature.

$$\text{Maintenance dose} = \frac{(0.16\ \text{L/min})\,(7\ \text{mg/L})\,(1\ \text{min})}{(0.82)\,(1)}$$

$$\text{Maintenance dose} = 1.4\ \text{mg/min}$$

The procainamide concentration should be checked in approximately 20 to 24 hours after the rate change. The active metabolite of procainamide, *N*-acetyl procainamide, also must be monitored.

## CASE 2

A 68-year-old man was admitted to the SICU following right femoropopliteal bypass graft surgery. Vital signs were stable with a mean arterial pressure of 85 mm Hg. The patient weighed 75 kg and had a body surface area of 1.6 m$^2$. His history included two myocardial infarctions 12 months and 5 years prior to admission. The patient's medications prior to surgery included insulin, enteric-coated aspirin, oral isosorbide, and diltiazem. His surgical history included a three-vessel coronary artery bypass procedure done 8 months earlier. One hour after admission to the SICU, the patient's blood pressure fell, and the following hemodynamic parameters were obtained:

| BP | MAP | P | CO | CI | PCWP | SVR | UO | Hb | $FIO_2$ | $PaO_2$ | $PaCO_2$ | pH | $HCO_3^-$ |
|---|---|---|---|---|---|---|---|---|---|---|---|---|---|
| 91/50 | 63 | 108 | 2.7 | 1.7 | 22 | 1450 | 25 | 11 | 0.6 | 109 | 41 | 7.32 | 20 |

The CXR results were consistent with pulmonary edema.

- *What is your assessment of the patient's hemodynamic state? How would you manage the patient to improve cardiac output and perfusion to vital organs?*

With a cardiac index (CI) of 1.6 L/min/m$^2$, a pulmonary capillary wedge pressure (PCWP) of 22 mm Hg, and a stroke volume of 25 ml, the patient is in acute cardiac failure following surgery. It would be appropriate to obtain an ECG and serial cardiac enzyme analyses to rule out perioperative myocardial infarction (MI).

Replacement of preload, afterload reduction, and administration of inotropic agents, alone or in combination, may improve cardiac function.

The patient's PCWP is already 22 mm Hg, and the CXR film shows signs of pulmonary edema. Additional preload probably would not be beneficial.

A vasodilator would be of benefit in this situation because of the patient's elevated PCWP and systemic vascular resistance (SVR). Lowering the PCWP and SVR would improve cardiac performance at a lower filling pressure. However, the patient already has a low mean arterial pressure (MAP) of 63 mm Hg, and there is a risk of further reducing MAP with a vasodilator. The consequent decrease in blood pressure, especially in diastole, may worsen myocardial ischemia.

An inotropic agent would be of benefit by increasing the stroke volume of the heart and improving the CI. However, inotropes increase myocardial work and oxygen demand by elevating contractility, systolic wall tension, and potentially heart rate. An appropriate approach would be to initiate an inotrope; if a reasonable MAP is established a vasodilator may be added to further improve cardiac output (CO), if necessary.

A dopamine infusion is started at 4 μg/kg/min and titrated to 9 μg/kg/min over the next 2 hours.

- *What are the physiologic effects of dopamine? Is the plan described here an appropriate dosing regimen?*

At doses of 4 to 10 μg/kg/min, the inotropic effect of dopamine is directly achieved through stimulation of beta-1 adrenergic receptors and indirectly done through release of norepinephrine, which improves cardiac performance. In low doses of 1 to 3 μg/kg/min, dopamine also stimulates dopaminergic receptors in the renal and splanchnic vascular beds to improve blood flow. At doses >10 to 15 μg/kg/min, dopamine stimulates alpha-adrenegic receptors, and an elevation in SVR with a reduction in renal blood flow occurs. The increase in SVR also limits CO.

An appropriate dose of dopamine would be one that elicits both the beta-1 inotropic effect and the vasodilating dopaminergic effect. The starting dose of 3 to 4 μg/kg/min should provide the desired receptor response. The infusion rate can be titrated by 1 to 2 μg/kg/min every 20 to 30 minutes until the desired hemodynamic outcome or, in this patient, a dose of 10 μg/kg/min has been reached. The desired outcome would be an improvement in the CI to at least 2.5 L/min/$m^2$, an MAP of at least 70 to 75 mm Hg, a reduced PCWP, increase in urine output to at least 0.5 ml/kg/hr, and a heart rate <110 beats/min. The hemodynamic responses to dopamine are highly variable; the hemodynamic variables must be checked at each new steady infusion rate, and the lowest effective infusion rate should be used.

The following hemodynamic measurements were obtained while the patient received a dopamine infusion at 9 μg/kg/min for 30 minutes:

| BP | MAP | P | CO | CI | PCWP | SVR | UO | Hb | $FIO_2$ | $PaO_2$ | $PaCO_2$ | pH | $HCO_3^-$ |
|---|---|---|---|---|---|---|---|---|---|---|---|---|---|
| 116/63 | 80 | 130 | 3.9 | 2.4 | 20 | 1460 | 35 | 11 | 0.6 | 110 | 38 | 7.38 | 20 |

- *Has the dopamine infusion been of benefit to the patient?*

The CI has improved somewhat, and the MAP has improved; however, the heart rate has increased significantly, and the SVR and PCWP have not changed. The urine output is still marginal. In this patient the administration of dopamine has improved the CI via a chronotropic effect rather than via increased contractility. Myocardial work has increased dramatically for the improvements obtained.

Attempts at reducing the heart rate and still maintaining the CI and perfusion pressure by decreasing the dopamine infusion rate proved to be unsuccessful. The physician initiated dobutamine, and the patient was weaned to 1 to 3 μg/kg/min dopamine in an attempt to improve the CI with less chronotropic effect.

- *What are the hemodynamic effects of dobutamine? What is its mechanism of action? Does dobutamine offer any advantages in hemodynamic response for this patient?*

The inotropic activity of dobutamine is a result of direct stimulation of beta-1 adrenergic receptors. In addition, this agent stimulates beta-2 and alpha-1 receptors to a lesser degree. The stimulation by beta-2 and alpha-1 receptors tends to cancel each other and produce only minimal direct effects on SVR. Unlike dopamine, dobutamine does not release norepinephrine or stimulate dopaminergic receptors. In patients with cardiac failure, dobutamine in doses of 2.5 to 15 μg/kg/min increases CO and decreases PCWP and SVR. The reduction in SVR is thought to result from a reflex response to the increased CO rather than from direct arterial vasodilation. Dobutamine also may be less chronotropic than dopamine, but the effect on heart rate is not predictable. The effectiveness of dobutamine at decreasing PCWP and SVR balances the increase in myocardial oxygen consumption that is caused by increased contractility and heart rate.

Dobutamine would offer several potential advantages over dopamine in this patient with elevated SVR and PCWP and excessively high heart rate. Dopamine tends to increase these variables, whereas dobutamine tends to decrease them or cause no change. Dobutamine is a better inotropic agent in the patient with depressed CO, elevated PCWP and SVR, mild hypotension, and concurrent cardiac ischemia.

A dobutamine infusion was started at 2.5 μg/kg/min and titrated to 8 μg/kg/min, and the dopamine was decreased to 3 μg/kg/min with the following results:

| BP | MAP | P | CO | CI | PCWP | SVR | UO | $FIO_2$ | $PaO_2$ | $PaCO_2$ | pH | $HCO_3^-$ |
|---|---|---|---|---|---|---|---|---|---|---|---|---|
| 120/62 | 81 | 112 | 4.4 | 2.8 | 16 | 1300 | 65 | 0.5 | 112 | 38 | 7.41 | 25 |

- *Have the addition of dobutamine and the reduction in dopamine been beneficial for the patient? Would amrinone be an appropriate alternative?*

The CI has been improved with dobutamine. Other effects include reductions in heart rate, SVR, and PCWP. The increase in perfusion pressure and the decrease in afterload, preload, and heart rate will improve the myocardial oxygen supply/demand ratio. Signs of improved systemic perfusion include a lessening of acidosis and improved urine output. The improved renal function may be secondary to the low-dose dopamine with improved renal perfusion.

Amrinone is a positive inotropic agent and vasodilator that acts by raising intracellular concentrations of cyclic adenosine monophosphate through inhibition of phosphodiesterase with a resultant modulation of intracellular calcium. It does not act on adrenergic receptors. Administration of amrinone to patients with severe heart failure results in a significant increase in CO and reduction in preload, SVR, and pulmonary vascular resistance. Heart rate and blood pressure usually are not altered. However, high infusion rates have caused tachycardia and hypotension. Amrinone should be used with caution in patients with hypotension, thrombocytopenia, and restrictive cardiomyopathies. Although dobutamine and amrinone have similar hemodynamic properties, dobutamine generally produces a larger increase in the CI. A trial of amrinone would have been appropriate in this patient if the dobutamine had not proven beneficial in improving CO or if drug-induced tachycardia had developed.

The patient's condition improved with dobutamine administered at 8 μg/kg/min and dopamine given at 3 μg/kg/min, and it remained hemodynamically stable.

- *With clinical stability, how should the patient be weaned from inotropic support?*

Both dopamine and dobutamine have an elimination half-life of approximately 2 to 3 minutes and can be tapered rapidly. When vasoactive agents are being tapered, time must be allowed for the patient to clearly show a response to the new lower dose before weaning is continued.

The dobutamine dosage could be reduced by 1 to 2 μg/kg/min every 30 to 60 minutes, and the dopamine could be kept at 3 μg/kg/min for its renal perfusion effect. After each step of the taper, hemodynamic measurements should be made. It would be appropriate to keep the PCWP between 12 and 18 mm Hg, MAP at 70 to 80 mm Hg, HR $<$110 beats/min, and the CI $>$2.5. On discontinuation of the dobutamine, the dopamine can be tapered.

## CASE 3

A 63-year-old man underwent surgical removal of his gallbladder without complication and was admitted to the SICU. He had a history of hypertension that was treated with metoprolol

(Lopressor) 50 mg orally bid and furosemide 80 mg orally qd. The patient also had chronic renal insufficiency (serum creatinine concentration 2.3 mg/dl). The patient weighed 80 kg preoperatively and had a body surface area of 1.8 $m^2$. On arrival in the SICU, the patient had the following hemodynamic profile:

| P | BP | MAP | UO | CO | CI | SVR | Hb | PCWP |
|---|---|---|---|---|---|---|---|---|
| 95 | 170/115 | 133 | 50 | 4.3 | 2.4 | 2500 | 11 | 10 |

- *What is your assessment of the patient's hemodynamic state?*

The patient is hypertensive. His SVR is elevated significantly, and the CO is low for a postoperative patient. The low CI is probably the result of an elevation in afterload and possibly a low preload. The patient should be assessed for adequate management of pain and anxiety to prevent further contribution to an elevated sympathetic tone.

The elevated blood pressure requires prompt treatment to reduce the work of the heart and to improve CO.

The patient was started on a nitroprusside continuous infusion at 0.3 μg/kg/min titrated to 2.5 μg/kg/min over 2 hours. The patient also received two fluid boluses of 250 ml of 5% albumin during this period. The following hemodynamic profile then was obtained:

| P | BP | MAP | UO | CO | CI | SVR | Hb | PCWP |
|---|---|---|---|---|---|---|---|---|
| 80 | 125/70 | 88 | 80 | 5.5 | 3 | 1080 | 10 | 13 |

- *Why was nitroprusside an appropriate agent to use? What other parenteral antihypertensive agents would be appropriate? Which oral antihypertensive agent should be instituted after the patient's blood pressure is controlled?*

Nitroprusside is a vasodilator of both the arterial and venous vasculature with a prominent effect on the arterial side. Therefore it reduces SVR along with blood pressure. Clearly, the patient demonstrated an elevated SVR, and nitroprusside should be effective in reducing blood pressure.

Preload also will be affected. Unless adequate fluid is given to compensate for the increase in venous pooling, the CO will fall or remain unchanged. Nitroprusside has a rapid onset and short duration of action, which makes it an ideal agent for treatment of acute hypertension. Since nitroprusside is administered by continuous infusion, it is possible to obtain smooth control of blood pressure. Possible thiocyanate toxicity secondary to nitroprusside is a concern in this patient because of his renal insufficiency. However, toxicity is rarely seen if the infusion rate is kept $<3$ μg/kg/min and therapy is limited to 72 hours or less.

Nitroglycerin is also a vasodilator with rapid onset and short duration of action, and it is administered by continuous infusion. Its predominant site of action is on the venous system. In the case of this patient, substitution of nitroglycerin for nitroprusside may have lowered the CO since the PCWP was in the low normal range.

Nitroglycerin would be a better choice than nitroprusside if the patient developed signs of myocardial ischemia. Nitroprusside may shunt coronary blood flow away from ischemic areas, whereas nitroglycerin improves flow to ischemic areas. Postoperative administration of nitroglycerin may be superior to the use of nitroprusside in cardiac surgery patients.

Labetalol, a parenteral alpha-1 blocker with nonspecific beta-blocker activity, would be a useful agent in this patient since he was receiving a beta-blocker prior to surgery. Labetalol's alpha-1 blockade will further lower SVR and blood pressure. This agent will cause a greater reduction in blood pressure than a pure beta-blocker such as propranolol would. Labetalol can be instituted via intravenous bolus administration or as a continuous intravenous infusion.

If the patient had contraindications to the use of agents with beta-blocker activity, such as a history of asthma or severe heart failure, intravenous administration of hydralazine, which has a fairly rapid onset of activity, would be appropriate. Hydralazine reduces SVR through direct relaxation of arterial smooth muscle. This drug can cause reflex tachycardia that may exacerbate ischemia in patients with coronary artery disease.

There are a number of oral antihypertensive agents that could be used as a substitute for the parenteral agent. Frequently, restarting the antihypertensive drugs that the patient was taking prior to surgery would be sufficient. However, some patients will require the addition or substitution of a different oral agent to maintain blood pressure control and allow weaning from the parenteral drug. Some of the more useful oral antihypertensive drugs that could be used are captopril, nifedipine or nicardipine, and labetalol. Oral labetalol would be a good substitute for metoprolol in this patient since it has beta-blocker activity.

# PART THREE

# *PATHOPHYSIOLOGIC CONDITIONS*

# SECTION 1 *Central Nervous System*

# CHAPTER 11

# *Evaluation of the Comatose Patient*

Martha A. Fehr • David S. Knopman

## CASE 1

A 60-year-old woman underwent orthotopic liver transplant because of end-stage primary biliary cirrhosis. On hospital day 3, she was unable to sleep. On day 4, she was disoriented regarding time and place. On day 5, she was found unresponsive. Her blood pressure was 170/117 mm Hg, pulse was 84 beats/min, and respirations were Cheyne-Stokes in type and 16/min. Pupils were pinpoint and reacted equally to light. Oculocephalic and oculovestibular responses were absent. Corneal reflexes also were absent. The extremities were flaccid with symmetrical stretch reflexes and bilateral flexor withdrawal responses to painful stimulation on the lower extremities. The toes were upgoing bilaterally.

- *What is your evaluation of the patient at this time?*

Coma in the setting of liver transplantation can occur for a number of reasons. The neurologic findings in this case are consistent with pontine level dysfunction and are more suggestive of a structural/anatomic cause of coma than a metabolic one.

The differential diagnosis includes pontine hemorrhage or infarction and central pontine myelinolysis. Other possibilities include cyclosporin toxicity, which can occur alone or with hypomagnesemia or hypocholesterolemia. Metabolic encephalopathy also should be ruled out but is less likely.

Initial evaluation should include a CT scan of the head to rule out pontine hemorrhage. An area of decreased attenuation consistent with either central pontine myelinolysis or cyclosporin toxicity may or may not be seen on the CT scan. If the initial CT scan of the head shows no hemorrhage, MRI may be helpful in ruling out these other possibilities.

Serum electrolytes, calcium, magnesium, phosphorus, liver enzymes, ammonia, BUN, creatinine, coagulation studies, cholesterol, and cyclosporin serum concentrations should be obtained.

This chapter can be studied in conjunction with *Essentials of Surgical Critical Care,* edited by Jerome H. Abrams and Frank B. Cerra (St. Louis: Quality Medical Publishing, Inc., 1993), Chapter 16.

Acute management is directed toward maintaining adequate airway and ventilation and correcting any metabolic abnormalities discovered. Hypertension is treated to bring blood pressure into the normal range. In this case the initial BP was 170/117. The target for antihypertensive therapy is 140 to 160 systolic over 80 to 90 diastolic. The use of mannitol has no place in this setting.

Results of the CT scan of the head were normal. MRI of the head showed an area of increased T2 signal in the pons and in the cerebral white matter. Serum sodium concentration was normal. Other laboratory values were normal with the exception of creatinine at 3.5, cholesterol at 76, and cyclosporin at 805 ng/ml. The immunosuppressant medications were adjusted. Over the next 10 days the patient's neurologic status gradually improved, and on hospital day 15 she was alert and moving all extremities. A repeat MRI scan showed resolution of the white matter changes.

The patient's liver function then deteriorated rapidly because of a subacute rejection. On day 17, while awaiting a second transplant, the patient suddenly slumped to the right and became unresponsive. Examination showed the BP to be 210/120 and the pulse was 90. The patient was intubated. The left pupil was dilated to 8 mm and fixed. The right pupil was 3 mm and reactive. The right side was flaccid, and the left side showed spontaneous decerebrate rigidity.

- *What is your assessment and your first course of action?*

The sudden onset of severe change in neurologic status is indicative of a catastrophic intracranial event. The right hemiplegia and the left dilated pupil indicate a left hemisphere space-occupying lesion with herniation. In this situation the most likely cause is an intracerebral hemorrhage. Hyperventilation should be instituted immediately. In addition, mannitol 1 g/kg body weight should be given intravenously. While these acute measures are being instituted, blood should be sent for measurement of CBC with platelet count and for coagulation studies. Disseminated vascular coagulation should be ruled out. Neurosurgery consultation should be obtained for possible immediate neurosurgical decompression. A CT scan of the head should be obtained when the patient is stable enough to be transported. Despite these efforts, the patient remained comatose and subsequently died.

## CASE 2

A 58-year-old man with hypertension and atherosclerotic cardiovascular disease underwent emergency coronary artery bypass graft. Postoperatively, he developed seizures involving the left arm and face. These seizures were described as intermittent twitching, beginning in the left hand and subsequently spreading to the left side of the face. The twitching would last 2 to 3 minutes with each occurrence. The patient was arousable and able to move his right side on command, but he could not control the left-sided twitching. A loading dose of phenytoin was administered, and no further clinical seizures were reported. However, the patient was noted to have decreased spontaneous movement of the left arm.

On examination, BP was 140/82 mm Hg and pulse was 80 beats/min. The patient was intubated. On neurologic examination, the patient was able to nod appropriately to questions and follow commands. Cranial nerve examination revealed a left central seventh nerve palsy. Left upper extremity strength was 3/5, and strength was 5/5 in the other extremities. The deep tendon reflexes were diminished in the left arm and normal in the other extremities. The toes were downgoing. Results of a CT scan of the head were normal.

Over the next 3 days, the strength in the patient's left arm gradually improved. The neurologic examination at that time showed a mild left central seventh palsy and a mild pronator drift on the left.

- *How would you assess the need for long-term anticonvulsant therapy in this patient?*

Postoperative focal seizures in patients undergoing cardiac surgery can occur for different reasons. They are commonly the result of embolic events. Emboli may be of cardiac origin. Microembolization related to the bypass machine also can occur, although it more often presents with diffuse mental status changes than with focal neurologic problems. Patients requiring cardiac surgery also may have preexisting subclinical cerebrovascular disease, and seizures may arise in a region of previous infarct. Intracranial hemorrhage is seen less often and, in a case such as this one would be unlikely, given the rapid recovery of neurologic function. Metabolic derangement, such as hypoglycemia, also can present with focal seizures and should be ruled out.

The character of the seizures described in this case is consistent with simple partial status epilepticus. The initial management is to control the seizures and then to determine the cause.

In this case, after the seizures were controlled, the patient had a residual mild left hemiparesis. This finding may represent a transient phenomenon, a so-called postictal Todd's paralysis, or, more likely, may represent a cerebrovascular accident. The mild degree of neurologic deficit is more suggestive of an embolic stroke rather than a thrombotic one.

Evaluation of the patient should include an EEG, which can demonstrate focal slowing that is suggestive of a structural abnormality and aid in ruling out subclinical seizure activity. The results of initial CT scan of the head were normal, a common occurrence in early infarction. The CT also can give normal results in the case of small embolic infarcts. An MRI of the head may demonstrate an area of infarct not seen on the CT scan.

Ultrasound cardiography is indicated to rule out the presence of a thrombus. This test will help in assessing the risk for further events and aid in deciding about the need for long-term anticoagulation. Carotid ultrasound examination also should be performed to rule out carotid source of emboli. The remainder of the evaluation should include CBC with platelet count, coagulation studies, and electrolyte concentrations, including glucose, calcium, magnesium, phosphorus, liver enzymes, BUN, and creatinine.

In terms of deciding the need for long-term anticonvulsant therapy, one must weigh the risk of recurring seizures resulting from an isolated embolic event; in the absence of permanent structural abnormality or persistent epileptiform activity on the EEG, the probability is small. In this situation, after the patient has recovered from his acute illness, the anticonvulsant medication can be discontinued safely. If, in the course of the evaluation, evidence of a structural abnormality is noted or persistent epileptiform activity on an EEG is recorded, then the patient may indeed need long-term anticonvulsant therapy.

This patient continued to show gradual improvement with virtual resolution of the left-sided deficits over 1 month's time. Results from a follow-up MRI scan of the head were normal. The EEG at that time also gave normal results. The phenytoin was discontinued, and no further seizures have been reported.

CHAPTER 12

# Seizures

Fernando Torres

## CASE 1

Three weeks after having been discharged, a 44-year-old woman was readmitted to the hospital because of seizures. On her previous admission, she had had subtotal resection of a large parasagittal meningioma complicated by malignant brain edema intraoperatively. A ventriculoperitoneal shunt was placed 2 weeks after surgery to decompress the craniotomy wound. The bone flap had been left out. The patient reported some nausea and vomiting. A productive cough appeared 4 days prior to admission. Focal seizure activity was noted the day before the patient's present admission to the neurosurgery service. The head and eyes turned to the right. No lip-smacking or extremity movements were noted. Seizures continued, and the patient became disoriented and confused, with short-term memory loss. Both seizures and mental status seemed to improve in the afternoon but worsened in the evening. The patient was receiving liquid phenytoin.

The patient's phenytoin level on the day of admission was 11. Her temperature had been going up and down, with two temperature spikes in the past 24 hours. Medications were phenytoin 350 mg liquid orally at night, heparin 5000 subcutaneously q 12 hr, ferrous sulfate 325 mg tid for anemia, folate 1 mg daily, and 1 multivitamin daily along with ibuprofen 600 mg orally tid prn.

Physical examination on admission revealed an obese woman with BP of 118/76, pulse of 100 beats/min, and respiratory rate of 16/min. A right temporoparietal craniotomy wound was healing well. The brain under the bone defect was soft and not bulging. Auscultation of the lungs demonstrated decreased, tubular breath sounds in the right base.

On neurologic examination, the patient was alert but disoriented. She followed commands slowly and inconsistently. Her speech was slow but without suggestion of aphasia. Extraocular movements were normal, but there was an obvious gaze preference to the right. The head tended to be kept turned to the right as well. A left facial palsy of central type was noted. The left upper extremity showed marked weakness, and the lower extremities showed mild spasticity, more pronounced on the left. Sensory examination was unreliable because the patient could not cooperate. Hyperreflexia of left extremities and bilateral Babinski's signs were noted.

A CT scan of the head showed no significant changes from the scan taken 1 week earlier: 6 to 7 mm subdural effusion on the left, causing no mass effect. There was no evidence of hydrocephalus, intracerebral hemorrhage, or infarction.

This chapter can be studied in conjunction with *Essentials of Surgical Critical Care,* edited by Jerome H. Abrams and Frank B. Cerra (St. Louis: Quality Medical Publishing, Inc., 1993), Chapter 17.

It was clear that a change in the patient's mental status had occurred since it had been normal 2 days before the present admission. Seizures had been reported, which suggested left frontal lobe onset. A CXR film revealed a right lower lobe infiltrate.

> A loading dose of phenytoin was administered, and the shunt was tapped, showing patency. Cloudy fluid was extracted, and the pressure was normal.
>
> The patient had repeated episodes of confusion with deviation of the eyes to the right. An EEG showed focal right frontotemporal slowing and very frequent focal electrical seizures in the left occipital area, spreading to all areas and associated with eye deviation to the right. In spite of the addition of lorazepam and carbamazepine, the seizures continued and the patient became obtunded. Antibiotics were administered.

Continuous monitoring with a cerebral function monitor (CFM) was started 2 days after admission in view of the comatose state, and continued seizures were recorded on daily EEGs. Very frequent seizures continued to be recorded on the CFM until 5 days after admission. At that time an EEG showed a markedly abnormal record with focal slowing and spikes in the right frontal area. The record showed no seizures, but there was no electrical reactivity to various kinds of stimuli.

The patient started to regain consciousness 2 days after the seizures became controlled. She continued to receive phenytoin and carbamazepine. Blood levels of anticonvulsants were high, with phenytoin at 30 μg/ml and carbamazepine at 12 μg/ml. Antibiotics also were given for pulmonary infection and meningitis. As the patient regained consciousness and started following commands consistently, she was weaned from the respirator.

Two weeks after admission to the neurosurgery service, the patient remained conscious with normal mental status. No further seizures occurred. Left hemiplegia and nystagmus were present. The patient was transferred to physical medicine and rehabilitation while continuing to take anticonvulsants, which were now at therapeutic blood concentrations. The prognosis was still considered guarded.

## CASE 2

> A 78-year-old man was transferred to a university coronary care unit from his local hospital, where he was admitted for left-sided chest pain of approximately 24 hours' duration. Apparently his admitting ECG showed inferior changes and atrial fibrillation, although cardiograms were not sent with the patient. The day after admission, creatine phosphokinase concentration peaked to 2263; no isoenzymes were sent for analysis. A CXR film apparently showed the possible presence of a left lower lobe infiltrate. The patient's temperature was 101° F. The patient developed an inferior myocardial infarction (MI) and did well until the morning of day 3 after admission, when he was found to have Cheyne-Stokes respirations and to be unresponsive to pain. Medications given at admission were digoxin 0.25 mg qd, quinidine 200 mg q 6 hr, dipyridamole 75 mg bid, furosemide 40 mg qd, and enteric-coated aspirin 2 tablets qid. The patient was allergic to penicillin.

The patient was admitted to the coronary care unit with a presumed inferior MI that was 3 days old and a new cerebrovascular accident. A CT scan of the head without contrast enhancement revealed a large infarct in the left middle cerebral artery distribution and no evidence of hemorrhagic infarct. A portable ultrasound cardiogram revealed a motion abnormality of the inferior wall. No mural thrombus was seen in the left ventricle. The left atrium was of borderline size.

Laboratory results at admission were Hb, 15.6; WBC count, 19,900 with 92% polymorphonuclear leukocytes; prothrombin time, 14.3; and platelet count, 288,000. Electrolytes were within normal limits, and creatinine was 1.6. The CXR film was poor but showed no evidence of infiltrate.

The patient was seen in consultation by the neurology consultant, who agreed with admission diagnoses and recommended that anticoagulants not be administered.

Overnight the patient reverted to atrial fibrillation with a slow ventricular response. At one point the systolic BP dropped to 80 mm Hg. Infusion of fluids raised the BP to 118/65. The patient then remained cardiovascularly stable. He had no evidence of ventricular ectopy. His ECG was stable overnight, and the decision was made to transfer him to the neurology service.

On examination in the neurology ICU, the patient was comatose. His temperature was 102.8° F rectally, respiratory rate was 22, with occasional Cheyne-Stokes respirations, pulse was 102 beats/min and irregularly irregular, and BP was 110/70. No peripheral edema was noted. When the patient's eyes were opened, the gaze was noted to be conjugate and to the left, but with full and conjugate extraocular movements on doll's head maneuver. Pupils were equal in size, round, and reactive to light. Fundi were benign. The neck was supple, with negative Kernig's and Brudzinski's signs. Diffuse rhonchi were heard over the lung fields. No murmurs, rubs, or gallops were heard. There was approximately 4 cm of jugular venous distention, without audible bruits. The abdomen was benign, with guaiac-negative stool on rectal examination. The patient was not arousable by any degree of deep pain or other stimulation. Corneal reflexes were bilaterally present. The right nasolabial fold was decreased, with a slight right labial droop. The gag response was intact. The patient was diffusely hyporeflexic, except for normal deep tendon reflexes of the right patella and both ankles, with downgoing left toe and equivocal upgoing right toe and negative Hoffman's signs bilaterally. The patient's right side was flaccid. The left upper extremity showed rare spontaneous movements and intermittently showed a resting "pill-rolling" tremor, with no movements of the left eye.

At the time of transfer to the neurology service, a CXR film showed a heart size at the upper limits of normal, which was difficult to evaluate since the film was a portable anteroposterior view, with a light left lower lobe infiltrate and right midlung infiltrate or atelectasis. A repeat cranial CT scan without contrast enhancement showed a large infarction in the left temporoparietal region, with diffuse cerebral atrophy. An ECG showed atrial fibrillation with a rate just above 100, with Q waves, ST-segment elevation, and T-wave inversion inferiorly.

- *What are the main diagnostic problems in this case at this time?*

The patient was considered to have had a large left hemispheric infarction, in the setting of a recent inferior MI. Echocardiography ruled out apparent mural thrombi or valvular vegetations as a source of possible emboli but did show a global mild decrease in left ventricular performance with a motion abnormality of the inferior wall.

With brainstem function intact as far as testable, there was no apparent explanation for the coma. Bilateral hemispheral infarctions could cause this state, but there was no evidence of right cerebral involvement. The coma was first thought to be secondary to unrecognized and presumably brief hypotension and/or hypoxia. A CT scan of the head was obtained without the use of intravenous contrast medium. Acute hemorrhage is usually visible on unenhanced CT scan. Thrombotic strokes generally do not enhance until at least 7 days have elasped. Sufficient information is usually obtained, however, and patients will not be subjected to the risk of intravenous contrast medium if an unenhanced CT scan is obtained at this time.

> An EEG performed at the bedside was reported as showing: "Marked abnormality with diffuse irregular slowing, more on the left. There were also frequent pseudoperiodic left parietal temporal spike bursts, which at times evolved into electrical seizures that became sometimes generalized, without clinical change." In view of the ongoing seizures, diazepam was injected intravenously. The EEG seizure activity showed decrease in frequency and duration after a 1 mg injection. After the second milligram, the seizures stopped, although interictal pseudoperiodic spikes continued to appear. The patient opened his eyes and moved his left arm and leg spontaneously. He seemed to look around but appeared aphasic.

In view of the dramatic change in the EEG and the awakening of the patient from a state of coma, it was decided to give him a loading dose of phenytoin. A total dose of 1400 mg of phenytoin was given intravenously within 30 minutes (about 50 mg/min), with the ECG and BP monitored. Phenytoin was then continued at a dose of 600 mg/day administered through the feeding tube, and a blood level of 12 μg/ml was achieved and maintained. The CFM was connected at the time of the initial EEG, and monitoring was continued to ensure that the patient would not have nonconvulsive seizures. Since the patient's state of consciousness did not change and no seizures were recorded on the CFM, monitoring was discontinued after 5 days.

The patient continued to be conscious but sleepy and aphasic. He showed no evidence of extension or reinfarction of the myocardium. Normal sinus rhythm was maintained by chemical conversion of digoxin and quinidine.

At the time of discharge, it was recommended that the patient remain on therapy with digoxin 0.25 mg qd per feeding tube, quinidine 200 mg q 6 hr per feeding tube, cimetidine 300 mg q 6 hr per feeding tube, antacid (Mylanta II alternating with Alternagel) 15 ml per feeding tube qid, phenytoin 350 mg q AM and 300 mg q PM per feeding tube, and heparin 5000 U subcutaneously q 12 hr. It was recommended that, with a recent increase in phenytoin from a total daily dose of 600 to 650 mg for a mildly subtherapeutic level of 9, the phenytoin concentration be rechecked several days after the patient's arrival home. In addition, continuous physical therapy was recommended for the patient's right hemiparesis.

# CHAPTER 13

# *Head Injury*

Eric S. Nussbaum

## CASE

A 24-year-old unhelmeted and intoxicated man was thrown from his motorcycle after being struck by a car. At the scene, the paramedics noted that he was unresponsive with equal, reactive pupils and a blood pressure of 110/50. The man's respirations were shallow, and he was intubated after immobilization of the cervical spine with a hard collar.

On arrival at the emergency department, the patient was hemodynamically stable with a heart rate of 96, blood pressure of 120/72, and oxygen saturation of 92%. He had bilateral equal breath sounds. The patient's eyes opened only with vigorous stimulation, his pupils were 4 mm in diameter, equal, and reactive. He withdrew his left arm and leg to pain but would not move his right side. A right femoral venous line was started, and an open left tibiofibular fracture with exposed bone was noted. The patient was ventilated at a rate of 16, and 50 g of mannitol was administered by the emergency room physician. Serum electrolyte concentrations were normal, and the hemoglobin was 12.6.

A head CT scan revealed a small left subdural hematoma with diffuse swelling and mild effacement of the left ventricular system. No midline shift was present. The abdominal CT scan was normal. The neurosurgical service elected observation of the patient's neurologic progression rather than evacuation of the hematoma at this time. Since a long orthopedic procedure was planned for repair of the fractures, a ventricular drainage catheter was inserted for intracranial pressure monitoring. The initial pressure was 24 mm Hg.

Several points concerning the initial care of this head trauma patient deserve emphasis. The first steps in the assessment of all trauma patients, including those with head injury, are the same. An adequate airway is established to ensure ventilation and to afford protection from aspiration. Hemodynamic stability is quickly assessed. Physical examination to evaluate breath sounds and pulses is essential. For example, a patient with a tension pneumothorax and an intracranial hematoma requires treatment for the pneumothorax before the hematoma can be addressed. In addition, the spine is assumed to be injured until proven otherwise, especially in a patient with altered sensorium from head trauma.

A preliminary neurologic examination should include checking the pupils, eye-opening, and motor and verbal responses. Patients with a Glasgow Coma Scale score <13 or with focal neurologic deficit should have a head CT scan. Even patients with milder head trauma also may require scanning. At this point neurosurgical consultation should be requested.

This chapter can be studied in conjunction with *Essentials of Surgical Critical Care,* edited by Jerome H. Abrams and Frank B. Cerra (St. Louis: Quality Medical Publishing, Inc., 1993), Chapters 5, 11, and *18*. Italicized number indicates the main chapter reference.

Until a head CT scan can be obtained, hyperventilation provides a simple, effective method to control intracranial pressure (ICP) in the intubated patient. The resultant hypocarbia causes cerebral vasoconstriction and diminishes the ICP. The ideal partial pressure of carbon dioxide ($Pco_2$) remains controversial, but a value <25 mm Hg makes the risk of ischemia too high. $Pco_2$ of 25 to 30 mm Hg is typically used in patients with severe head trauma, and 30 to 35 mm Hg is used in milder cases.

The osmotic diuretic mannitol is an effective agent in controlling ICP. It is typically administered as a bolus of 1g/kg body weight or as a continuous infusion. In hypotensive patients, mannitol may worsen hypovolemia and therefore should be used with great care. Steroids, which were once frequently used after head injury, have proven to be of no demonstrable benefit, and their use for such injury is not indicated.

Direct monitoring of ICP remains controversial. Conventionally, any head injury patient in whom one cannot follow a neurologic examination or whose neurologic status is so poor that deterioration would be difficult to detect deserves ICP monitoring. In the case of this patient, neurologic examination was impossible for the extended period of time that he was paralyzed and sedated for the orthopedic procedure. The subdural hematoma could have expanded and the patient could have suffered transtentorial herniation while in a state of general anesthesia, with no one realizing the situation until hours later. The use of a ventricular catheter to measure ICP, instead of a subarachnoid screw or an intraparenchymal monitor, provides the added advantage of allowing the drainage of CSF to further lower the ICP.

Eight hours later, the patient was brought to the SICU. On initial assessment, the patient was still sedated and paralyzed and had an ICP of 14 mm Hg. Laboratory values included: Na, 133 mEq/L; K, 3.6 mEq/L; Hb, 7.8 g/dl; PT, 18.4 sec; PTT, 39.2 sec; and lactate, 1.4 mmol. A central venous catheter was inserted, maintenance IV fluid was switched to normal saline at 75 ml per hour, potassium replacement was given, and packed RBCs and fresh frozen plasma were transfused. The muscle relaxants were discontinued.

Over the next 3 hours, with elimination of the muscle relaxants, the ICP began to rise. When suctioning was done, the patient opened his eyes and demonstrated flexor posturing. The ICP was now 28 mm Hg, the $Pco_2$ was 34 mm Hg, and the serum osmolality was 279. The patient was sedated with codeine and midazolam, mannitol was again administered, and the ventilatory rate was increased. Over the next 20 minutes, the ICP fell to 16 mm Hg.

After head trauma, careful attention must be paid to maintaining normal electrolyte values. Patients with such injury often receive the diuretic agent mannitol and are also at risk for the development of SIADH. Therefore frequent sodium and potassium checks are indicated. In addition, it is important to rapidly correct abnormalities in coagulation studies to prevent delayed hemorrhage. All patients with intracranial hematomas are typically given a loading dose of an anticonvulsant agent because they have increased risk for seizures. Since attempts are made to minimize fluid administration to prevent cerebral edema, many patients will require central venous monitoring or a pulmonary artery catheter to ensure adequate systemic hemodynamic resuscitation.

In general, ICP should be maintained at <20 mm Hg. In this case, the $Pco_2$ was 34 mm Hg, a value that suggests further hyperventilation might be of benefit. Similarly, the serum osmolality was low, a finding that supports the use of additional mannitol. If the serum osmolality were higher than 315, additional mannitol probably would not be useful. Sedation is also helpful in controlling ICP; in severe cases, paralysis with sedation or barbiturate coma may be required to decrease ICP. Treatment of head injury by induction of barbiturate coma should be undertaken only with expert consultation.

Over the next 24 hours, the ICP remained below 12 mm Hg. Routine follow-up head CT scan revealed no change in the size of the hematoma. The patient began to follow simple commands and opened his eyes spontaneously. The $P_{CO_2}$ was allowed to slowly return to normal over 48 hours. With a $P_{CO_2}$ of 41, the ICP remained low and the ventriculostomy was removed. A nasal feeding tube was inserted, and enteral nutrition was begun.

On hospital day 5, the patient was noted to be less responsive, not following commands, and had a generalized tonic-clonic seizure. A head CT scan revealed diffuse swelling and no change in the subdural hematoma. Laboratory values were notable for a sodium concentration of 122 mEq/L and a dilantin concentration of 6. The sodium was slowly corrected over 24 hours, and a repeat bolus of dilantin was administered. The patient returned to his prior neurologic status.

The head trauma patient remains a challenge, even after the acute phase of injury has been treated successfully. Nutritional support is important since the patient probably will not be eating normally for a long time. Electrolyte values must be carefully monitored and maintained in the normal range. In this case hyponatremia most likely precipitated the seizure. Gradual correction of the sodium concentration is important to avoid pontine damage. It is important to remember that patients who deteriorate neurologically, even when apparently stable several days after injury, should undergo head CT scanning.

Aggressive diagnostic and therapeutic interventions at the earliest signs of neurologic deterioration are the key to successful management of the head trauma patient.

# CHAPTER 14

# *Spinal Cord Injury*

**Eric S. Nussbaum • Leslie A. Sebring**

## CASE

An 18-year-old unbelted passenger in a motor vehicle accident was thrown through the windshield of his car and struck the pavement 15 feet away. At the accident scene, he was reported to be unconscious. His blood pressure was 100/60, and his heart rate was 60. He was intubated after stabilization of the cervical spine in a hard collar.

On arrival at the emergency department, the patient's blood pressure was 90/65, heart rate was 55, and oxygen saturation was 95%. He appeared warm and well-perfused. A femoral venous line had been established and 2 L of lactated Ringer's solution had been infused. The patient was being ventilated at a rate of 14 breaths/min. Breath sounds were equal bilaterally, eyes were open, pupils equal and reactive to light, and the patient was able to follow simple commands. After 5 minutes, his blood pressure was 85/45, and a neosynephrine infusion was started. Blood pressure rose to 100/60.

On closer neurologic inspection, the patient demonstrated a flaccid paralysis in the lower extremities. He had no movement in the upper extremities but did shrug his shoulders. A Foley catheter was placed and returned 750 ml of urine. Rectal tone was absent, and all reflexes, including the bulbocarvernosus, were absent. Lateral cervical spine x-ray examination revealed bilateral facet dislocation at the C6-C7 level with 50% subluxation of C6 on C7. Diagnostic peritoneal lavage was negative.

As with any trauma victim, the initial care of this patient includes ensuring an adequate airway, ventilation, hemodynamic stability, and immobilization of the spine. In the unconscious trauma patient who is hypotensive, diagnostic peritoneal lavage can be performed rapidly and in a setting where chest and abdominal injuries can be managed immediately. If the patient has no source of hemorrhage, and if the blood pressure cannot be supported with volume loading, pressors may be necessary. Usually the hypotensive trauma victim who does not respond to such aggressive fluid administration is typically in profound hemorrhagic hypovolemic shock. In hypovolemic shock the blood pressure is low and the heart rate is high as a consequence of reflex tachycardia. The patient is peripherally vasoconstricted, with shunting of blood to the central circulation. The other possibility that must be considered in the hypotensive trauma patient is spinal cord injury resulting in neurogenic or spinal shock. Unlike the patient with hemorrhagic shock, such patients are hypotensive with an inappropriately low heart rate and appear well perfused peripherally as a result of loss of the sympathetic tone after disruption of the spinal cord sympathetic fibers.

---

This chapter can be studied in conjunction with *Essentials of Surgical Critical Care*, edited by Jerome H. Abrams and Frank B. Cerra (St. Louis: Quality Medical Publishing, Inc., 1993), Chapters 5 and *19*. Italicized number indicates the main chapter reference.

The spinal cord injury patient is, therefore, peripherally vasodilated and may be surprisingly slow to respond to fluid resuscitation. For this reason pressors may be needed to temporarily reverse the hypotension and to maintain an adequate blood supply to the injured spinal cord. The spinal cord injury patient is typically initially areflexic and hypotonic.

In the trauma patient, the spinal cord should be assumed to be injured until proven otherwise. Numerous reports have documented iatrogenic neurologic deterioration after manipulation of the spinal cord injury patient without proper spine immobilization.

A neurosurgical consultation was obtained. The patient was placed in Gardner-Wells traction. He was started on a steroid protocol consisting of a bolus of 30 mg/kg of methylprednisolone over 15 minutes, followed by 5.4 mg/kg/hr for the next 23 hours. An $H_2$-receptor antagonist was started simultaneously. The patient was taken in traction to the CT scanner. CT examination of the head was normal. An attempt to perform closed reduction of the dislocation with serial incrementation of the traction weights was unsuccessful, and the patient was taken to the operating room and underwent an open reduction procedure.

Neurosurgical consultation should be obtained immediately on admission for any cervical spine injury. The goal of treatment for such injuries is rapid stabilization of the spine and reduction of any subluxation. While the specific treatments of the different cervical spine fractures are detailed and beyond the scope of this presentation, there are several basic points that must be remembered.

Typically, three views of the cervical spine are required to be certain that no osseous injury has occurred. These include an anteroposterior view, an open-mouth odontoid view, and a lateral view that includes the cervicothoracic junction. If a bony injury is identified, one must consider its immediate vs. late potential for stability, but most importantly one must decide if the spine is currently stable. Is a hard cervical collar sufficient? Does the patient require halo brace fixation? Will an operation be necessary to establish stability?

Recently, the above steroid protocol has been shown to improve outcome from spinal cord injury when administered within 8 hours of injury. Although it may only improve the neurologic function by one spinal level, this additional function may mean the use of the hands for a paraplegic patient.

Five hours later, the patient was brought to the SICU. Initial laboratory values included: Na, 138 mEq/L; K, 3.1 mEq/L; Hb, 11.7 g/dl; Hct, 34.8%; lactate, 0.9 mmol; PT, 17.5 sec; and PTT, 41.2 sec. The blood pressure was 110/65, and the heart rate was 75. The patient was intubated with low-dose neosynephrine infusion. A central venous line was inserted, fresh frozen plasma was transfused, and potassium was replaced. Subcutaneous administration of heparin was begun, and elastic hose and compression stockings were applied.

On the following day, parenteral nutrition was begun. The patient remained hemodynamically stable. The physical therapy department was consulted to initiate range of motion exercises. Over the next 72 hours, repeated attempts to wean the ventilatory support failed because the patient was unable to clear his secretions. The nurses began to suction thick secretions, and a right middle-lobe infiltrate appeared on the CXR film. These findings were accompanied by an increase in the WBC count and a low-grade fever. Sputum cultures grew a coagulase-negative *Staphylococcus* bacterium that was sensitive only to vancomycin. This antibiotic therapy was initiated, and the patient was started on nebulizer treatments, percussion, and drainage every 4 hours, as well as hourly suctioning.

One of the major challenges in the management of the spinal cord injury patient is the meticulous care necessary to prevent secondary complications. Such patients are particularly prone to pulmonary and urinary infections that require aggressive therapy. Routine blood, urine, and sputum cultures for fever spikes are important in identifying the source of infection. Careful pulmonary toilet must be encouraged, and early removal of indwelling catheters and lines is emphasized. Frequent turning of the patient or special rotating beds are essential to prevent decubitus ulcers. A bowel regimen should be instituted.

With respect to pulmonary complications, it should be noted that the sources of innervation to the diaphragm are the C3, C4, and C5 roots. A high cervical spine injury can result in paralysis or dysfunction of the diaphragm muscle and can disrupt the innervation of the intercostal muscles. Patients with such injuries may be ventilator-dependent for life. It is also important to recognize that a spinal cord injury can ascend several levels after admission. Consequently, even a C6-C7 lesion may affect diaphragmatic function. Fluoroscopic examination of diaphragmatic motion may provide important information regarding such dysfunction.

> By day 13, the pulmonary infiltrate had resolved, and the fever had disappeared. The WBC count had returned to normal. Fluoroscopy of the diaphragms was normal. On day 28, a tracheostomy was performed to facilitate pulmonary toilet. The patient was successfully weaned from the ventilator 1 week later, and his family was instructed regarding intermittent bladder catheterization. The patient was transferred to an inpatient rehabilitation facility for further care.

The recovery of the spinal cord injury patient is often quite slow and presents numerous frustrating setbacks. Aggressive rehabilitation is essential. The ultimate outcome from spinal cord trauma should be decided not days but months after initial injury, and every effort must be concentrated on meticulous care to prevent secondary complications from hindering such recovery.

## SECTION 2 *Cardiovascular Function*

# CHAPTER 15

# *Altered Cardiac Physiology*

**Vivian L. Clark • James A. Kruse • Richard W. Carlson**

### CASE 1

A 70-year-old man with a remote history of an anteroseptal myocardial infarction presented with acute hematemesis. A nasogastric tube was inserted, and bright-red blood was aspirated from the stomach. Vital signs were: pulse 110 $min^{-1}$; BP, 110/90 mm Hg; respiratory rate 14 $min^{-1}$; and temperature 37.2° C (99° F). Hb was 9.4 g/dl, and hematocrit was 28%. The patient was admitted to the SICU, where a central venous catheter was inserted, revealing a central venous pressure measuring 6 mm Hg. The patient was given 1500 ml of lactated Ringer's solution and two units of packed RBCs. Shortly after receiving the second unit of blood, the patient complained of chest pain and developed respiratory distress requiring endotracheal intubation. An ECG showed sinus tachycardia, Q waves in leads $V_1$-$V_4$ consistent with prior anteroseptal myocardial infarction, and downsloping ST-segment depression in leads II, III, and aVF. A CXR film showed pulmonary vascular congestion. A bedside echocardiogram revealed a dilated left ventricle with anteroseptal akinesis and inferior hypokinesis. Global left ventricular ejection fraction was estimated at 30%.

- *What is your assessment?*

This case illustrates the special difficulty posed by fluid resuscitation in patients with underlying systolic dysfunction and diminished cardiac reserve. The ECG demonstrated changes consistent with previous myocardial infarction (MI) plus changes compatible with acute ischemia. This is corroborated by the echocardiographic findings of regional wall motion abnormalities and reduced ejection fraction. The patient's acute decompensation was probably precipitated by a combination of factors, including underlying coronary disease, systolic dysfunction from a previous MI, and acute ischemia. The acute ischemia could have been precipitated by the increase in heart rate and systemic vascular resistance (SVR) attributed to the initial hypovolemia and anemia. Vigorous volume loading probably resulted in excessive increases in left ventricular

This chapter can be studied in conjunction with *Essentials of Surgical Critical Care,* edited by Jerome H. Abrams and Frank B. Cerra (St. Louis: Quality Medical Publishing, Inc., 1993), Chapters 2 and *20.* Italicized number indicates the main chapter reference.

filling pressure and cardiogenic pulmonary edema. Although the patient's central venous pressure (CVP) remained normal, CVP is frequently a poor reflection of left ventricular filling pressure in patients with underlying cardiovascular disease.

Following intubation, the patient's BP was 120/90 mm Hg, and the pulse was 120 $min^{-1}$. Rales over both lung bases and an $S_3$ gallop were heard on auscultation. A pulmonary artery (PA) catheter was inserted and revealed the following hemodynamic values: CVP, 8 mm Hg; right ventricular pressure, 36/8 mm Hg; pulmonary artery pressure (PAP), 36/28 mm Hg (mean 31); pulmonary capillary wedge pressure (PCWP), 26 mm Hg; cardiac output (CO), 3.5 $L \cdot min^{-1}$; cardiac index (CI), 1.9 $L \cdot min^{-1} \cdot m^{-2}$; SVR, 3900 $dyne \cdot sec \cdot cm^{-5} \cdot m^2$; and pulmonary vascular resistance (PVR), 210 $dyne \cdot sec \cdot cm^{-5} \cdot m^2$.

The clinical and hemodynamic findings are typical of acute left ventricular decompensation. PCWP is markedly elevated, despite the fact that CVP is only mildly increased. The CI also is reduced despite the elevated PCWP. SVR is markedly increased because of the reflex vasoconstriction that commonly occurs with systemic hypoperfusion and helps to maintain blood pressure.

The patient was treated with morphine sulfate, topical nitroglycerin, and intravenous furosemide. His chest pain and ST-segment depression subsided, he had diuresis of 1000 ml, and there was no further evidence of active GI bleeding. Subsequent hemodynamic findings were: pulse, 94 $min^{-1}$; BP, 115/80 mm Hg (mean 92); CVP, 8 mm Hg; PAP, 30/20 mm Hg (mean 23); PCWP, 18 mm Hg; CO, 4.5 $L \cdot min^{-1}$; CI, 2.5 $L \cdot min^{-1} \cdot m^{-2}$; SVR, 2700 $dyne \cdot sec \cdot cm^{-5} \cdot m^2$; and PVR, 160 $dyne \cdot sec \cdot cm^{-5} \cdot m^2$.

The patient's condition improved with pharmacologic therapy aimed at preload reduction (furosemide, nitrates, and morphine) and treatment of underlying ischemia (nitrates). Continued treatment with antianginal therapy is indicated, and after resolution of the acute GI problem, further evaluation of the patient's underlying coronary disease also may be indicated.

## CASE 2

A 64-year-old man had an unremarkable medical history except for symptoms of prostatism. Following transurethral resection of the prostate, he developed fever and mental confusion. Vital signs were: pulse, 128 $min^{-1}$; BP, 88/60 mm Hg (mean 69); respiratory rate, 24 $min^{-1}$; and temperature, 39.1° C (102.4° F). Laboratory findings included a WBC count of 22,500 $mm^{-3}$ and a blood lactate concentration of 4.5 $mmol \cdot L^{-1}$. Blood and urine cultures were obtained, empiric intravenous antibiotic treatment was initiated with administration of a cephalosporin and an aminoglycoside, and the patient received a dose of monoclonal antiendotoxin antibodies. He was transferred to the SICU and underwent bedside PA catheterization, which revealed: CVP, 3 mm Hg; PAP, 28/13 mm Hg (mean 18); PCWP, 7 mm Hg; CO, 7.4 $L \cdot min^{-1}$; CI, 4.4 $L \cdot min^{-1} \cdot m^{-2}$; SVR, 1200 $dyne \cdot sec \cdot cm^{-5} \cdot m^2$; PVR, 200 $dyne \cdot sec \cdot cm^{-5} \cdot m^2$, left ventricular stroke work index (LVSWI) 29 $g \cdot m \cdot m^{-2}$; and right ventricular stroke work index (RVSWI), 7 $g \cdot m \cdot m^{-2}$.

- *What further therapeutic measures should be considered?*

The low PCWP suggests that left ventricular preload is not optimal and that volume loading is in order.

The patient received 1000 ml of isotonic crystalloid and 500 ml of 6% hetastarch during the next 2 hours. The CVP and PCWP increased to 7 and 9 mm Hg, respectively, and the CI increased to 4.9 L · $min^{-1}$ · $m^{-2}$, but the BP remained unchanged, and urine output during the last hour was only 20 ml.

- *Should a vasopressor infusion be administered?*

Although treatment with a catecholamine such as dopamine could be initiated at this point as a temporizing measure to raise blood pressure, the filling pressures are probably still suboptimal for a patient with sepsis and perfusion failure. Therefore additional fluid should be administered to further raise the PCWP in an attempt to increase CO.

Additional isotonic fluid was administered at 20 ml · $min^{-1}$ while PCWP was monitored at 10-minute intervals. After 60 minutes, the PCWP reached 14 mm Hg, BP rose to 105/70 mm Hg, and the pulse decreased to 116 $min^{-1}$. The fluid challenge was stopped, and a repeat hemodynamic profile was obtained. The CI was 5.6 L · $min^{-1}$ · $m^{-2}$; SVR, 1000 dyne · sec · $cm^{-5}$ · $m^2$; LVSWI, 44 g · m · $m^{-2}$; urine output, 30; and partial pressure of oxygen ($PaO_2$), 76 mm Hg with supplemental oxygen ($FIO_2$ 0.4). A CXR film revealed evidence of early diffuse bilateral infiltration.

Intravenous fluids were continued to provide maintenance and replacement of ongoing losses, and infusions of low-dose dopamine (3 μg/kg/min) and dobutamine (5 μg/kg/min) were started. The PCWP remained at the same level, BP and urine output improved further, and a repeat CI done 2 hours later was 5.9 L · $min^{-1}$ · $m^{-2}$. Blood lactate concentration decreased to 2.3 mmol · $L^{-1}$, and $PaO_2$ remained stable.

Further fluid administration proved to be of benefit as evidenced by the increase in the CI and improvement of other physiologic variables. Since pulmonary vascular congestion does not usually occur on a cardiogenic basis with PCWP values below 18 to 20 mm Hg, the physicians considered an additional cautious fluid challenge to determine whether the CI would respond further to increases in preload. However, because (1) the present PCWP is known to be optimal for many patients with sepsis, (2) the patient showed clinical and hemodynamic evidence of improvement at this level of PCWP, and (3) the CXR and blood gas findings suggested the possibility of early adult respiratory distress syndrome, the PCWP of 14 mm Hg was judged to be adequate, and further fluid challenge was not done. The decrease in blood lactate concentration and improvement in urine output were indicative of favorable effects of the catecholamine infusions on systemic perfusion.

Blood and urine cultures subsequently showed growth of *Escherichia coli* sensitive to the administered antibiotics. Four days later the patient was afebrile, his sensorium was improved, blood pressure was stable without catecholamines, and there was no worsening of his respiratory status. The patient progressed to complete recovery.

## CASE 3

A 35-year-old man with no significant medical history came to the emergency department complaining of dyspnea and pleuritic chest discomfort, which had developed during the previous 3 to 4 days. The chest pain had become significantly worse on the day of admission. The patient stated that he had been involved in an altercation several days earlier, during which he was stabbed in the chest with a barbecue fork, but he did not seek medical attention at that time.

On physical examination, the patient's pulse was 120 $min^{-1}$ and regular, respiratory rate was 22 $min^{-1}$, and temperature was 38° C (100.4° F). BP was 96/78 mm Hg, but the systolic BP was noted to fall to 85 mm Hg during inspiration. The patient's neck veins were distended to the angle of the jaw. The lungs were clear. Cardiac examination revealed diminished heart tones, and no murmur, gallop, or friction rub was noted. Two small puncture wounds were noted over the parasternal precordium.

- *What further diagnostic tests are indicated?*

This patient presents with a history of penetrating thoracic trauma and hypotension. The initial differential diagnosis includes cardiac perforation, tamponade, coronary artery laceration, tension pneumothorax, and mediastinitis. The physical findings of pulsus paradoxus, distended neck veins, and diminished heart sounds suggest pericardial tamponade.

An ECG showed sinus tachycardia with reduced QRS voltage. A CXR film showed questionable enlargement of the cardiac silhouette and no pulmonary vascular congestion. An arterial line and PA catheter were inserted. Mean arterial pressure was 84 mm Hg; CVP, 22 mm Hg; PAP, 34/24 mm Hg (mean 28); PCWP, 25 mm Hg; and CI, 1.9 L · $min^{-1}$ · $m^{-2}$. The SVR was 2600 dyne · sec · $cm^{-5}$ · $m^2$, and the PVR was 130 dyne · sec · $cm^{-5}$ · $m^2$. A bedside echocardiogram revealed a moderate-sized pericardial effusion and right atrial and right ventricular inspiratory collapse.

Following the administration of intravenous fluids and supplemental oxygen, the patient appeared clinically improved, and the BP and CI increased modestly. The patient was taken to the operating room, where exploration of the thorax revealed a moderate amount of bloody pericardial effusion containing a few blood clots. After removal of only 50 ml of fluid, the BP increased to 120/80 mm Hg and the pulse rate declined to 90 $min^{-1}$. No active bleeding was identified. A pericardial window was performed, and the patient had an uneventful recovery.

The presence of pericardial fluid confirmed by echocardiography, in conjunction with equalization of right atrial pressure (RAP), diastolic PAP, and PCWP, supports the diagnosis of pericardial tamponade as the cause of shock in this patient. The marked hemodynamic improvement after removal of only a small quantity of pericardial fluid is typical of tamponade and also confirms the diagnosis.

# CHAPTER 16

# *Acute Myocardial Infarction*

Robert E. Cunnion • Steven M. Hollenberg

## CASE 1

A 63-year-old woman with a history of heavy smoking and labile hypertension was admitted for elective cholecystectomy. On anesthetic induction, she developed frequent premature ventricular contractions, and her BP fell from 150/90 to 110/60. The procedure was cancelled. On awakening, the patient became diaphoretic and complained of chest discomfort. Her pulse was 110 beats/min, BP 160/100, and respiratory rate 22/min; she had no murmurs, gallops, or rales. A 12-lead ECG showed 2 mm ST-segment elevation and peaked T waves in leads $V_1$ and $V_2$. A peripheral IV catheter was inserted and nasal oxygen was administered. The patient was monitored with an ECG, a pulse oximeter, and an automatic BP cuff.

- *What initial pharmacologic management is appropriate?*

The immediate goal is pain relief, to reduce sympathetic tone and reduce myocardial oxygen demand. This can be accomplished with sublingual nitroglycerin (0.4 mg q 5 min × 3 doses), followed by aliquots of morphine sulfate (2 mg IV q 5 min), until relief is obtained or hypotension supervenes. It would also be appropriate at this time to have the patient suck or chew an aspirin tablet. Lidocaine should be given only for symptomatic dysrhythmias.

After 30 minutes, the patient had received 3 sublingual nitroglycerin tablets, 6 mg of morphine, and 1 aspirin tablet. Her chest pain, though diminished, persisted. The patient's pulse was 100 beats/min and BP was 150/90; her lungs were clear. Her ECG still showed 2 mm ST-segment elevation in $V_1$ and $V_2$.

- *What therapy is indicated?*

It had become clear that the patient was having an acute anteroseptal myocardial infarction (MI) and not just a prolonged anginal episode. There were no contraindications to thrombolytic therapy; streptokinase 1.5 million U should be given intravenously over 1 hour. In addition, an intravenous nitroglycerin infusion should be started at 10 μg/min and titrated to reduce systolic pressure by 10% to 20%.

Acute beta-blockade (e.g., metoprolol 5 mg IV q 5 min × 3 doses) should be considered if tachycardia and chest pain persist, but beta-blockers should not be given if there are signs of heart failure.

The patient's chest discomfort and hypertension subsided with the intravenous nitroglycerin; her pulse decreased to 70 after a total of 15 mg of intravenous metoprolol. As the streptokinase

This chapter can be studied in conjunction with *Essentials of Surgical Critical Care,* edited by Jerome H. Abrams and Frank B. Cerra (St. Louis: Quality Medical Publishing, Inc., 1993), Chapters 20 and *22.* Italicized number indicates the main chapter reference.

infusion was completed, she had several short runs of asymptomatic nonsustained ventricular tachycardia. The ECG showed return of the ST segments in $V_1$ and $V_2$ to baseline, with T-wave inversion and early evolution of Q waves.

- *What steps should be taken now?*

Until this point, the patient has had an uncomplicated Q-wave infarction. The streptokinase and other interventions are intended to minimize infarct size. Reperfusion dysrhythmias are common with thrombolytic therapy. The patient should remain in a monitored setting and have serial ECGs and cardiac enzyme determinations. The intravenous nitroglycerin can be tapered after 24 hours. Heparinization may not be needed following streptokinase. Aspirin and beta-blockers should be taken as long-term secondary prevention. Acute cardiac catheterization is not needed unless ischemia recurs.

## CASE 2

A 65-year-old man with diabetes underwent colonic resection for a Dukes' B adenocarcinoma. On postoperative day 2, he became short of breath. Examination revealed a regular pulse of 120 beats/min, BP of 88/50, respiratory rate of 30, and an $S_3$ gallop and bibasilar rales. ABG analysis while the patient was receiving 2 L/min nasal oxygen showed 7.42/30/112/99%. A 12-lead ECG showed a left bundle branch block, a new development since admission.

- *What steps should be taken next?*

The constellation of ECG changes, acute left ventricular failure, and hemodynamic instability is very suggestive of MI; ischemia can be present without chest pain in individuals with diabetes. Pulmonary embolism is less likely. An embolism massive enough to cause hypotension ordinarily would cause more pronounced hypoxemia and would not ordinarily produce rales or a left bundle branch block. The patient should be transferred immediately to a monitored unit with an IV catheter, ECG monitoring, pulse oximetry, and an arterial line. Fluids can be given to raise the patient's blood pressure, but they must be used cautiously in the face of congestive heart failure. Diuretics, nitrates, and morphine sulfate are all relatively contraindicated by the low blood pressure. Patients whose infarctions are heralded by new-onset left bundle branch block do benefit from thrombolytic therapy, but this patient's recent surgery was an absolute contraindication. It would be exceedingly difficult to optimize the management of his fluids and inotropic agents without a pulmonary artery catheter.

A pulmonary artery catheter was placed. The hemodynamic measurements were:

| RA | RV | PA | BP | PCWP | CO | CI | SVRI |
|---|---|---|---|---|---|---|---|
| 10 | 39/5 | 38/25 | 88/50 | 21 | 3 | 1.5 | 2806 |

Dobutamine was started at 5 μg/kg/min, but the patient's BP drifted down to 78/48. There were no signs of ventricular septal rupture or acute mitral valve papillary muscle rupture.

- *What should be done next?*

The patient was developing cardiogenic shock, with hypotension, a low CI, and a high SVRI. The PCWP was already high; therefore additional fluid would be likely to exacerbate pulmonary edema without improving ventricular performance. Vasodilators, such as nitroprusside, might lower PCWP and increase CI but are impractical in the face of hypotension. Dobutamine might be titrated upward, but at the expense of increased myocardial oxygen demand and at the risk of infarct extension. The mortality for cardiogenic shock with pharmacologic treatment alone is >90%. Accordingly, an effort should be made to stabilize the patient with intra-aortic balloon counterpulsation, and he should undergo emergency coronary arteriography. Once the infarct-related coronary artery is identified, revascularization should be attempted immediately with angioplasty or coronary artery bypass grafting.

# CHAPTER 17

# *Hypertensive Emergencies*

John W. Hoyt

## CASE 1

After having an anterior communicating aneurysm clipped, a 39-year-old woman was admitted to the SICU for postoperative monitoring. The patient had been previously healthy, but 48 hours earlier she had suddenly developed the worst headache of her life. She sought care in the emergency department, where a CT scan of the head confirmed the diagnosis of ruptured subarachnoid aneurysm. Results from a lumbar puncture were positive. An arteriogram demonstrated a large aneurysm in the area of the anterior communicating artery with moderate vascular spasm. A regimen of nimodipine and intravascular volume loading was begun, and 2 days later the patient was taken to the operating room for craniotomy. The first postoperative BP in the SICU was 220/130, and the HR was 130. The patient was very agitated and thrashing about in bed. Anesthetic technique had been induction with sodium thiopental and muscle paralysis with vecuronium. Maintenance of anesthesia was accomplished with fentanyl, droperidol, nitrous oxide, and oxygen, with doses of vecuronium as needed by train-of-four neuromuscular monitoring.

Many neurosurgical patients develop hypertension and tachycardia in the postoperative period. Patients are particularly prone to hypertension after craniotomy for subarachnoid aneurysm. Areas of the brain may lose autoregulation after surgery, making hypertension a dangerous sequela. A substantial increase in blood pressure in the absence of autoregulation will increase cerebral blood flow and can worsen postoperative edema and elevate intracranial pressure. In this patient it was unclear whether the hypertension was primarily related to agitation or to the surgical procedure. After neurologic evaluation, it would be acceptable to try 50 to 100 μg of fentanyl intravenously to see if the patient is calmer and less hypertensive.

After a dose of fentanyl the patient was clearly less agitated but still arousable. Hypertension persisted (BP 200/120), as did tachycardia (HR 120). Further analgesia and sedation was not desirable because of concerns about clouding the neurologic examination, which continued to be as expected for the early postoperative period.

Control of blood pressure at this point would require the use of an antihypertensive agent. Since the starting heart rate was >110, a drug with beta-blocking properties would be helpful.

This chapter can be studied in conjunction with *Essentials of Surgical Critical Care*, edited by Jerome H. Abrams and Frank B. Cerra (St. Louis: Quality Medical Publishing, Inc., 1993), Chapters 20, 22, and *23*. Italicized number indicates the main chapter reference.

The patient had no history of reactive airway disease and did not have and never had had congestive heart failure. An agent with direct vasodilating properties such as hydralazine or nitroprusside might markedly reduce cerebral vascular resistance, increase cerebral blood flow, and elevate intracranial pressure. Considering the need to control heart rate, prevent reflex tachycardia, and avoid a direct vasodilating effect on the cerebral vasculature, labetalol seemed a good choice.

A starting dose of 5 mg of labetalol was given intravenously with no response in 5 minutes. The dose was increased to 10 mg, then 5 minutes later to 20 mg, at which time the BP was 190/110 and the HR 105. Three subsequent doses of 20 mg given 5 minutes apart reduced the BP to 170/90 and the HR to 85. The patient was resting comfortably after the fentanyl but was arousable by a normal neurologic examination.

Labetalol is a nonselective beta-blocker and a selective alpha-2-blocker that has about equal effects on blood pressure and heart rate. If doses effect a 25% reduction in blood pressure, one can expect about a 25% reduction in heart rate. Hypovolemic patients are very sensitive to this agent and can quickly become dangerously hypotensive. In order to protect against such hypotension, the starting intravenous dose should be 5 mg. This can be increased to 10 mg and then 20 mg when the patient's response to therapy has been determined. Labetalol does not increase cerebral blood flow and intracranial pressure, as nitroprusside and hydralazine have been demonstrated to do.

Thirty minutes after the last dose of labetalol, the patient's BP was 200/100 and the HR 105. There was no sign of agitation, but the patient complained of pain in the area of the incision.

Once again, a dose of intravenous fentanyl controlled the pain but failed to reduce the blood pressure. The patient was given another 20 mg of intravenous labetalol. A continuous infusion of labetalol was started at 30 mg/hr after the bolus dose. One hour later the BP was 170/85 and the HR 90. The infusion of labetalol was continued throughout the evening of the first postoperative day. Results of neurologic examination continued to be normal, and repeat CT scans of the head the next morning showed minimal postoperative edema and bleeding.

## CASE 2

After right carotid endarterectomy, the postoperative course for a 63-year-old diabetic man was notable for hypertension (BP 190/100) in both the recovery room and in the cardiovascular surgery stepdown unit. The patient had a history of hypertension controlled with diuretic alone (BP 140/70). Diabetes was managed with diet, and historically most of his blood glucose concentrations had been in the high 100s during the 15 years he had been known to have diabetes. In addition, the patient had a vague history of chest pressure that had never been evaluated by cardiac catheterization since his ECG was normal and he seemed to have no limitation of activity. The patient had nitroglycerin at home but used it only once or twice a week. He had smoked one pack of cigarettes per day since the age of 16, and his father died of a heart attack at the age of 53.

The carotid disease was found by auscultation of the neck during routine physical examination. A subsequent arteriogram revealed significant occlusions of both the right and left carotid arteries, but the right artery was more severe so it was chosen for the first surgical correction. The intraoperative course was managed anesthetically with a cervical plexus block and mild sedation using midazolam and fentanyl. Only 700 ml of fluid was given during the procedure. The patient lost 100 ml of blood but was awake most of the time and conversing with the nurse anesthetist and anesthesiologist. Intraoperative blood pressure was not a problem. At 2 AM the next day the patient was noted by the stepdown unit nurse to be short of breath, to complain of pressure in the chest, and to have basilar rales on auscultation of the chest. The surgical resident was called to evaluate the patient.

This patient belongs to a group of individuals who have a high likelihood of diffuse vascular disease; he was diabetic, smoked, had a family history of heart disease, and at a rather early age (63) had extensive carotid disease. More than likely, this patient had aortic, femoral, and coronary artery occlusions that were not evaluated in his preoperative visits because of minimal symptoms. In addition, his history of diabetes made his story of rare chest pressure very difficult to evaluate when, based on symptoms alone, one attempted to quantify the amount of coronary disease that might have been present. His postoperative BP was substantially above his normal levels, and it would appear that he was in a cardiac-decompensated state based on the impact of hypertension on a diseased cardiovascular system.

The surgical resident found the patient to have CHF and pulmonary edema. BP was 210/110 and HR 118. Obviously distressed, the patient was breathing 40 times per minute and was covered with perspiration. An ECG revealed ST-segment depression and T-wave inversion across the precordium. ABG analysis demonstrated a pH of 7.48, partial pressure of carbon dioxide ($Paco_2$) of 33 mm Hg, arterial partial pressure of oxygen ($Pao_2$) of 48 mm Hg on 4 L of nasal prong oxygen, which was started by the nurse when the patient initially complained of shortness of breath. The patient was transferred immediately to the SICU. An arterial catheter was inserted, which confirmed the previous blood pressure readings taken by an automated noninvasive blood pressure system. Pulse oximetry continued to demonstrate hypoxia with a 78% saturation. Shortness of breath worsened. Furosemide 40 mg and morphine 5 mg were given intravenously and a dose of nitroglycerin was administered sublingually. A 100% rebreathing oxygen mask replaced the nasal prong oxygen.

Appropriate first-line therapy for congestive heart failure and pulmonary edema was chosen. There was no clinical reason that this patient should be overloaded with fluid based on intraoperative and postoperative fluid management. The pulmonary edema must have been caused by cardiac ischemia secondary to hypertension. Ischemia changes the compliance of cardiac muscle and markedly increases left ventricular end-diastolic pressure (LVEDP) for a previously normal left ventricular end-diastolic volume. Elevated LVEDP will markedly increase pulmonary capillary wedge pressure, which represents a hydrostatic driving force to flood the interstitial space of the lung with fluid. This is a case of cardiogenic pulmonary edema, but of a left ventricular dysfunction type rather than a fluid-overload type. Furosemide is a pulmonary capillary vasodilator as well as a diuretic and, as a result, is good initial therapy in the management of pulmonary edema based on left ventricular dysfunction. Morphine has afterload-reducing properties, and nitroglycerin is a good preload reducer to lower the hydrostatic driving pressure in the pulmonary capillaries.

Fifteen minutes after initiation of therapy, the patient was less symptomatic. The pulse oximeter saturation was 88%, but the BP remained 195/105 and the HR was 115. A repeat ECG continued to demonstrate ischemia in the precordial leads. The patient noted about a 20% reduction in chest pressure. Enalaprilat 0.625 mg was given intravenously. Thirty minutes later, the BP was 185/98 and the HR 118. Chest pressure persisted.

Persistent chest pain and ischemia in the patient was now largely caused by tachycardia since the blood pressure was slowly coming under control. The tachycardia is sinus in nature and is compromising diastolic time, which is essential for blood flow to the myocardium to occur during diastole. In addition, the tachycardia increases the cardiac demand for oxygen, as does the residual hyptertension. Further correction of ischemia in this patient must address the issue of tachycardia.

> The surgical resident decided to lower the heart rate by using a cardioselective beta-blocker. Esmolol was started at 50 μg/kg/min, which reduced the HR to 105. This dose was subsequently increased first to 100 μg and then to 150 μg/kg/min, which reduced the HR to 90. BP was now 155/85, and the patient was free of chest pressure. The following morning, an ECG showed a complete resolution of the ischemic changes. Cardiac enzyme tests revealed a small increase in creatine phosphokinase-MB, reflecting a non–Q-wave myocardial infarction. The patient was monitored in the SICU for 3 more days. He was switched to oral metoprolol when the esmolol was stopped, and a regimen of diltiazem was started as both antihypertensive and anti-ischemia therapy. The patient was scheduled for further evaluation of his cardiovascular system.

The use of beta-blockers in the face of obvious left ventricular failure is always a difficult decision. This patient had persistent tachycardia, which was detrimental to the balance of myocardial oxygen supply and demand. He sustained a non–Q-wave myocardial infarction as a result of that imbalance. In this setting esmolol was a very good choice because it acts very quickly. If the use of a beta-blocker had further aggravated ventricular failure, the drug would have cleared the bloodstream within 10 to 20 minutes of discontinuing the infusion. This patient had good systolic function, as demonstrated by his hypertension, and there was no history of myocardial infarction, congestive heart failure, or low ejection fraction. Beta-blockers are usually well tolerated and ultimately very beneficial in such a setting because of their effect on myocardial oxygen supply/demand balance.

# CHAPTER 18

# *Cardiopulmonary Interactions*

Michael R. Pinsky

## CASE 1

A 34-year-old woman weighing 105 kg underwent a routine cholecystectomy for recurrent gallstones that were not responsive to lithotripsy. Her trachea was extubated postoperatively, and she was returned to her ward bed. In the ensuing 2 days, the patient complained of vague abdominal pain, nausea, and mild dyspnea. She received fluid support of normal saline with 5% dextrose at the rate of 125 ml/hr until she could start taking fluids orally. On postoperative day 2, the patient developed increasing epigastric pain, fever (temperature 39.5° C), tachycardia (HR 125, regular), nausea, and respiratory distress. ABG analysis revealed partial pressure of oxygen ($PaO_2$) of 55 mm Hg, partial pressure of carbon dioxide, ($PaCO_2$) of 30 mm Hg, and pH to be 7.48 while breathing 2 L oxygen by nasal cannula. A CXR film revealed bilateral lower lobe atelectasis and pleural effusions. CBC revealed leukocytosis with a left shift and a hematocrit of 34%. Serum amylase concentration was moderately elevated. All other blood chemistry results were normal.

The patient was given supplemental oxygen (40% by face mask), encouraged to breathe deeply and cough, and transferred immediately to the SICU, where blood cultures and a repeat ABG analysis were performed. Results of the ABG analysis revealed $PaO_2$ of 42 mm Hg, $PaCO_2$ of 45 mm Hg, and pH of 7.31. Vital signs were respiratory rate 32, temperature 39.5° C, BP 98 mm Hg/palpable by cuff, and pulse 125. Due to increasing agitation, central cyanosis, and presumed impending respiratory arrest, an attempt was made at endotracheal intubation with the patient awake, but without success. The patient was then sedated with midazolam, and tracheal intubation was done easily. The patient was then given positive-pressure ventilation with the following settings: tidal volume 1200 ml, frequency 15/min, fraction of inspired oxygen ($FIO_2$) 0.6 mm Hg, and positive end-expiratory pressure (PEEP) 5 cm $H_2O$.

Within minutes of the intubation, the patient became more unresponsive and profoundly hypotensive; BP was 60 mm Hg/palpable, and the pulse was thready at 150. Good breath sounds without wheezing were heard bilaterally. A portable CXR film demonstrated that the endotracheal tube was in proper position and that a significant amount of the atelectasis observed in the previous film had resolved. Repeat ABG analysis revealed a $PaO_2$ of 255 mm Hg, $PaCO_2$ of 25 mm Hg, and pH of 7.31. The tidal volume was reduced to 800 ml, a central intravenous access was obtained, and rapid fluid resuscitation with normal saline in 250 ml

This chapter can be studied in conjunction with *Essentials of Surgical Critical Care*, edited by Jerome H. Abrams and Frank B. Cerra (St. Louis: Quality Medical Publishing, Inc., 1993), Chapters 20, *24*, and 27. Italicized number indicates the main chapter reference.

boluses was performed. After approximately 1000 ml of normal saline had been infused, the patient's BP increased to 135/75 and the pulse decreased to 85. The metabolic acidosis resolved within 1 hour. The results of follow-up blood cultures were negative, and the patient was successfully extubated to 24% $FIO_2$ by face mask on the following day.

The patient demonstrated most of the detrimental effects of positive-pressure ventilation on venous return. The clinical course was one of postoperative atelectasis in a volume-depleted patient, made worse by her obesity and the nature of her operation, which required an upper abdominal incision. The patient's fluid requirements following recent abdominal surgery with third-space fluid loss, fever, and no oral intake resulted in a relatively hypovolemic state. Since she was obese, increases in lung volume increased intrathoracic pressure (ITP) more than in a nonobese patient, as a result of the added weight of the abdominal contents on the diaphragm. The mechanism is analogous to the effect of ascites on ITP. Furthermore, as documented by the repeat ABG analysis, the initial tidal volume delivered was too high, making ITP rise further. The choice of initial tidal volume settings, though based on body weight, should have been referenced to ideal body weight since the extra fat contributed little to metabolic demand.

Appropriate treatment of such a patient may include tracheal intubation if obtundation prevents the use of mask continuous positive airway pressure (CPAP). Hypotension, tachycardia, and worsening hypotension sedation and the clinical setting all suggest hypovolemia. Thus rapid and aggressive fluid resuscitation may be necessary in such patients to prevent a hypotensive crisis.

## CASE 2

A 65-year-old man weighing 65 kg and having history of severe chronic obstructive pulmonary disease due to tobacco abuse (125 pack-year exposure) developed acute hematemesis and syncope. Esophagogastroendoscopy documented an arterial bleeding site at the base of a duodenal ulcer. The patient underwent routine vagotomy and pyloroplasty, with oversewing of the ulcer, and was returned to the SICU intubated. Since the patient had a history of severe chronic obstructive pulmonary disease (forced expiratory volume [$FEV_1$]/forced vital capacity ratio = 0.25, $FEV_1$ = 900 ml), no attempt was made to wean him from mechanical ventilatory support on postoperative day 1. On postoperative day 2, the patient appeared hemodynamically stable, afebrile, and alert. ABG analysis revealed $PaO_2$ of 120 mm Hg, $PaCO_2$ of 35 mm Hg, and pH of 7.44 with an $FIO_2$ of 0.4, intermittent mandatory ventilation (IMV), tidal volume of 700 ml, and a frequency of 20.

Weaning was attempted by progressively decreasing the IMV frequency in five-breath increments every 4 hours as tolerated. Although the patient appeared comfortable with an IMV frequency of 15/min, when the rate was reduced further, he became agitated, tachypneic (respiratory rate 35/min), and tachycardic (sinus rhythm, pulse 125), with diffuse inspiratory and expiratory wheezes. Pulmonary arterial and radial arterial catheters were inserted and gave the following hemodynamic data, which were obtained at different levels of ventilator support.

| *Measurement* | *Rate (breaths/min)* | | |
|---|---|---|---|
| IMV | 20 | 15 | 10 |
| PEEP | 0 | 0 | 0 |
| $Pa_{O_2}$ | 120 | 115 | 85 |
| $Pa_{CO_2}$ | 35 | 37 | 67 |
| pH | 7.44 | 7.43 | 7.18 |
| RR | 20 | 25 | 35 |
| HR | 95 | 105 | 125 |
| Pra | 15 | 17 | 32 |
| Ppa | 35/18 | 36/20 | 56/35 |
| Ppao | 12 | 13 | 30 |
| Pa | 110/75 | 112/80 | 75/45 |

IMV was then continued in the patient at the frequency of 20/min and inhalational bronchodilator therapy was begun. The acute tachycardia, tachypnea, and elevations of right atrial pressure (Pra), pulmonary artery pressure (Ppa), and pulmonary artery occlusion pressure (Ppao) reversed over 1 hour. Afterward, the patient was placed on maintenance bronchodilator therapy and given supplemental levels of PEEP until pulmonary artery diastolic pressure (Ppa) increased. The tidal volume was decreased to 600 ml. These therapies resulted in the following ABG values: $Pa_{O_2}$ of 125 mm Hg, $Pa_{CO_2}$ of 48 mm Hg, and pH of 7.38. Repeat weaning from the lower tidal volume with 6 cm $H_2O$ PEEP allowed the patient to be extubated within 24 hours.

Patients with severe chronic obstructive pulmonary disease have an increased work-cost of breathing. Furthermore, their ability to exhale is time-limited, making air-trapping a risk when ventilatory rates are high. This patient was ventilated at too high an initial minute ventilation, which resulted in down-regulation of the acid-base status to a lower $Pa_{CO_2}$. The patient was unable to maintain that level of minute ventilation during weaning for two reasons. First, the work-cost of breathing was too high. Second, air-trapping caused by the high spontaneous ventilatory rate decreased respiratory muscle efficiency further and increased ITP. The result was an increase in intrathoracic vascular pressures caused by the increase in ITP. Note the diastolic equilibration of all pressures. Supplemental extrinsic PEEP to offset the auto-PEEP effect allows spontaneous ventilatory efforts to occur without large swings in ITP.

Therapies that limit hyperinflation will improve mechanical efficiency of the respiratory muscles and will prevent both increases in end-expiratory ITP and large swings in ITP during ventilation. Bronchodilator therapy, permissive hypercarbia, and supplemental extrinsic PEEP all function to achieve this goal.

# SECTION 3 *Pulmonary Function*

# CHAPTER 19

## *Acute Lung Injury*

Larry A. Woods • James P. Davison • Alan J. Cropp

### CASE 1

A 34-year-old man was the unbelted driver of a car that struck a bridge overpass head-on. Paramedics at the scene stated that the windshield was broken but the steering wheel was intact. The patient was awake, lethargic, and responding to questions, but he had no recollection of the accident. He was extricated from the car with adequate cervical spine and back immobilization. A 16-gauge IV catheter was placed, and normal saline solution was administered. The right leg was immobilized because of gross deformity.

In the emergency department, two 16-gauge IV catheters were placed, and lactated Ringer's solution was infused. The patient was found to be awake and alert, but still amnesic to recent events. Vital signs at the time were a pulse rate of 136, BP 95 mm Hg systolic, respiratory rate of 26, and a core temperature of 36.2° C (97.2° F). Physical examination revealed cool, moist skin. Multiple minor scalp lacerations were noted. Ears, nares, and pharynx were clear. Pupils were equal in size and reactive, and fundi were normal. Breath sounds were equal and clear. Pain was elicited over ribs 4-6 on the right. Heart sounds were normal. The abdomen was soft and nontender with normal bowel sounds. The right thigh was markedly swollen, as was the right calf. Angulation of the right lower leg at midcalf was noted. The skin was intact. Pulses were present but diminished in the right leg. There were no focal neurologic deficits. Nasogastric fluid and urine analyses were negative for blood. Results of the rectal examination were normal. Congo red stain of the urine showed no fat. Results of x-ray studies of the pelvis and the cervical spine and CT scans of the head and abdomen were negative. The CXR film was remarkable only for nondisplaced fractures of ribs 5 and 6 on the right. X-ray films of the right lower extremity showed angulated fractures of the femur, tibia, and fibula. An arteriogram of the right femoral artery showed a tear at the femoral fracture site. ECG showed only sinus tachycardia. Results of routine laboratory studies performed in the emergency department were essentially normal. The hemoglobin was 9 g, and the results of coagulation studies were normal.

---

This chapter can be studied in conjunction with *Essentials of Surgical Critical Care,* edited by Jerome H. Abrams and Frank B. Cerra (St. Louis: Quality Medical Publishing, Inc., 1993), Chapters 1, 2, 5, 18, *25,* and 27. Italicized number indicates the main chapter reference.

ABG analysis, with the patient breathing room air, showed a pH of 7.47, partial pressure of carbon dioxide ($PaCO_2$) of 32 mm Hg, and partial pressure of oxygen ($PaO_2$) of 54 mm Hg. The patient was placed on a 100% non-rebreather mask resulting in a rise of $PaO_2$ to 285 mm Hg and an $O_2$ saturation of 99%.

The patient was transfused in the emergency department with 3 units of packed RBCs and 4 L of crystalloid solution. The systolic BP increased to 110 mm Hg, and the pulse decreased to 110 beats/min. A pulmonary artery catheter inserted intraoperatively revealed a pulmonary capillary wedge pressure (PCWP) of 8 mm Hg. The patient was transfused with another 3 units of packed RBCs and an additional 4 L of crystalloid solution. The right femoral artery vascular repair and right femur open reduction proceeded uneventfully. Estimated surgical blood loss was 1200 ml, and urine output was 500 ml. The patient was taken to the SICU still intubated. Ventilator settings were synchronized intermittent mandatory ventilation (SIMV) 14, tidal volume 1000 ml, and fraction of inspired oxygen ($FIO_2$) 0.4.

Although the patient appeared stable at this time, certain cardiopulmonary variables were abnormal.

- *What are these variables? What factors should be considered in the care of this patient?*

First, the patient has suffered a head injury. Despite the negative results of the CT scan, he must be observed for any neurologic changes such as focal deficits or changes in mentation. Cardiac contusion is also a concern and may be evaluated by 2-D echocardiogram, which may demonstrate pericardial effusion or segmental wall motion abnormalities. Adequate tissue perfusion and oxygen delivery must be maintained while avoiding fluid overload or potential risk for oxygen toxicity.

The large incremental change in $PaO_2$ after institution of high concentrations of supplemental oxygen suggests ventilation/perfusion mismatch as a cause for the baseline hypoxemia. It must be kept in mind that this patient has three risk factors associated with acute lung injury: multiple long-bone fractures, multiple blood transfusions, and lung contusion. Arterial oxygen saturation must be continuously monitored or frequent ABG studies must be performed. A peripheral arterial catheter should be considered for arterial pressure monitoring and in anticipation of the need for frequent ABG measurements. If tachypnea and increased peak airway pressures occur, acute lung injury (ALI) should be suspected and the causes should be vigorously investigated.

Other factors to be considered in this patient's care are maintenance of adequate urine output through fluid and intravascular volume assessments. Observation for signs of continued bleeding and development of compartment syndrome as well as hypothermia should be considered. Pain management and nutrition are important considerations in the overall management.

Six hours postoperatively, the patient was awake and stable. Pain control was adequate by using intravenous narcotics every 1 to 2 hours. Vital signs at this time were BP 130/70, pulse 95 beats/min, respirations 22 on SIMV mode of 10 breaths/min. Pulse oximeter demonstrated a 97% saturation. The patient's increased respiratory rate was attributed to pain, and more intravenous morphine was administered. Over the next 4 hours, the respiratory rate climbed to 28 breaths/min, and the oxygen saturation decreased to 83%, despite an increase in $FIO_2$ to 70%. Plateau airway pressures increased to 30 cm $H_2O$ on the ventilator. ABG analysis showed a pH of 7.5, $PaCO_2$ of 28 mm Hg, $PaO_2$ of 52 mm Hg, and a saturation of 83%. CXR film revealed interstitial edema in three of four quadrants. The pulmonary artery catheter showed a mean pulmonary artery pressure (MPAP) of 25 mm Hg, PCWP of 12 mm Hg, and no changes in CO.

- *What is the lung injury score (Table 19-1)? What are the treatment goals?*

**TABLE 19-1** Components and Individual Values of Lung Injury Score*

| Components | Value |
|---|---|
| ***CXR examination*** | |
| No alveolar consolidation | 0 |
| Alveolar consolidation confined to one quadrant | 1 |
| Alveolar consolidation confined to two quadrants | 2 |
| Alveolar consolidation confined to three quadrants | 3 |
| Alveolar consolidation in all four quadrants | 4 |
| ***Hypoxemia score ($Pa_{O_2}/F_{IO_2}$)*** | |
| ≥300 | 0 |
| 225-299 | 1 |
| 175-224 | 2 |
| 100-174 | 3 |
| <100 | 4 |
| ***PEEP score (when ventilated)*** | |
| ≥5 cm $H_2O$ | 0 |
| 6-8 cm $H_2O$ | 1 |
| 9-11 cm $H_2O$ | 2 |
| 12-14 cm $H_2O$ | 3 |
| ≥15 cm $H_2O$ | 4 |
| ***Respiratory system compliance score (when available)*** | |
| ≥80 ml/cm $H_2O$ | 0 |
| 60-79 ml/cm $H_2O$ | 1 |
| 40-59 ml/cm $H_2O$ | 2 |
| 20-39 ml/cm $H_2O$ | 3 |
| ≤19 ml/cm $H_2O$ | 4 |
| The final value is obtained by dividing the aggregate sum by the number of components that were used. | |
| ***Lung injury*** | ***Score*** |
| None | 0 |
| Mild-to-moderate | 0.1-2.5 |
| Severe (ARDS) | >2.5 |

$Pa_{O_2}/F_{IO_2}$, arterial oxygen tension to inspired oxygen concentration ratio; PEEP, positive end-expiratory pressure.
*Modified from Murray JF, Matthay MA, Luce J, et al. An expanded definition of the adult respiratory distress syndrome. Am Rev Respir Dis 138:721, 1988.

The patient was developing severe ALI, as suggested by the lung injury score of >2.5. Hypoxemia refractory to increasing levels of inspired oxygen is consistent with intrapulmonary shunting. The patient should be managed with the assist control mode and positive end-expiratory pressure (PEEP). PEEP should be instituted at 5 cm $H_2O$ and raised in 2.5 to 5 cm $H_2O$ increments until an adequate level of arterial oxygenation is achieved ($Pa_{O_2}$ ≥60 mm Hg or $O_2$ saturation ≥90%).

As the levels of PEEP increase, risk for barotrauma increases. When changing to the assist control ventilator mode, a worsening of the respiratory alkalosis may occur secondary to increased minute ventilation. Sedation, with or without complete muscle paralysis, may be required to decrease minute ventilation and alleviate the respiratory alkalosis.

The ventilator was changed to an assist control mode. PEEP was added in increments of 5 cm $H_2O$ until satisfactory levels of both arterial oxygenation and inspired oxygen concentrations were achieved. This was found at a PEEP of 10 cm $H_2O$ and an $FIO_2$ of 50%. Arterial oxygenation rose to $PaO_2$ 78 mm Hg and saturation to 96%. CO decreased after institution of PEEP. A fluid bolus of 200 ml of normal saline solution returned this value to its original level. The patient remained intubated for the next three hospital days without further event. After showing marked improvement, the patient was weaned from the ventilator and extubated, and he recovered fully.

## CASE 2

A 65-year-old woman was brought to the emergency department after suffering a syncopal episode. She had complained to family members of dysuria and intermittent right-flank tenderness for the past week. For 2 days prior to admission, she had had fever accompanied by rigors. She was awake but lethargic in the emergency department. Initial vital signs included a pulse of 130 beats/min, systolic BP of 70 mm Hg, respiration of 30 breaths/min, and temperature of 102.6° F. The patient's skin was warm and dry without rash. Her pupils were equal in size and reactive, and her neck was supple. Breath sounds were equal and clear. Results of the cardiac examination were unremarkable. The abdomen was soft, mildly distended, and had decreased bowel sounds. Rectal examination showed no occult blood.

Two 16-gauge IV catheters were placed, and normal saline solution was rapidly infused. A WBC count of 26,000/$mm^3$ with a marked left shift was noted, as well as an Hb of 15 g/dl and a hematocrit of 46%. The platelet count was 240,000/$mm^3$. ABG analysis showed a pH of 7.3, $PCO_2$ of 24 mm Hg, $PaO_2$ of 65 mm Hg, and $HCO_3^-$ of 11.8 mEq/L with the patient breathing room air.

A CXR film was clear without cardiomegaly, and an ECG showed only sinus tachycardia. A Foley catheter was placed, and 100 ml of cloudy, foul-smelling urine was drained. The urine contained abundant WBCs and numerous Gram-negative bacilli.

- *What is your appraisal of the patient?*

The patient presented with clinical evidence suggesting septic shock. Patients with septic shock are at high risk for developing ALI, and early aggressive treatment is essential.

Therapy should include concurrent attention to the following: (1) rapid and aggressive fluid resuscitation and vasopressor support, (2) appropriate broad-spectrum antibiotic therapy, (3) end-organ evaluation and support, and (4) consideration for administration of antiendotoxin antibody.

Return of adequate intravascular volume without fluid overload is an essential first step in attempting to maintain hemodynamic stability. Therapy should be guided by central monitoring, utilizing a pulmonary artery catheter. Controversy exists as to the optimal fluid to use in restoring hemodynamic stability. Less colloid is required when compared to a similar amount of crystalloid infused to achieve the same hemodynamic endpoint and may be considered for use in this case. Recently a combination of hypertonic saline solution and albumin has been advocated, but current data do not support routine use of this regimen.

Broad-spectrum antibiotics should be started and adjusted when culture results are available. Of great importance is the administration of antibiotics as soon as possible after appropriate cultures are obtained. In recent studies antiendotoxin antibody, if given early, has demonstrated efficacy in reduction of morbidity and mortality in this patient subgroup. Corticosteroids are not indicated and actually may worsen prognosis. The use of NSAIDs and xanthine derivatives in sepsis is still investigational.

A two-antibiotic regimen was started in the emergency department. Three liters of crystalloid were infused with a notable increase in systolic BP to 90 mm Hg. Two liters per minute of oxygen via nasal cannula was administered, and the patient was transported to the SICU. Pulmonary and peripheral artery catheters were placed. Initial hemodynamic parameters were obtained: CO 5.84 L/min; MPAP 22 mm Hg; pulmonary capillary wedge pressure (PCWP) 9 mm Hg; mean arterial pressure 60 mm Hg; systemic vascular resistance (SVR) 708 dyne · sec · $cm^{-5}$. Urine output was 10 ml/hr. The serum lactate concentration was 5.9 mmol/L. Over the next 4 hours, 3.5 L of crystalloid and 500 ml of colloid was infused. Dopamine infusion at 5 μg/kg/min was started, and repeat measurements demonstrated an increase of CO to 8.4 L/min, MPAP to 32 mm Hg, and SVR to 692 dyne · sec · $cm^{-5}$. Urine output increased to 80 ml/hr. Serum lactate concentration decreased to 2.8 mM/L. Repeat ABG analysis on 2 L/min via nasal cannula were obtained: pH 7.38, $Pco_2$ 28 mm Hg, and $Po_2$ 58 mm Hg.

The hemodynamic improvement observed resulted from an increase in intravascular volume and adequate ventricular filling pressures. Improvements in CO, tissue perfusion, and oxygen delivery resulted in decreased anaerobic metabolism and lactate production. Adequate urine output was reestablished with hydration and a small dose of dopamine.

Although cardiac and renal function improved, the presence of early acute lung injury may be suggested by pulmonary hypertension and hypoxia. Early in the course of acute lung injury, the pulmonary hypertension is responsive to pharmacologic interventions such as vasodilators. However, vasodilator therapy has not been shown to affect outcome and may even worsen arterial oxygenation by increasing shunt fraction. Hypoxia in the absence of elevated left-side filling pressure should alert the physician to consider the early diagnosis and treatment of ALI and the further need for close monitoring of respiratory function and possible early intubation.

Cardiac and renal function remained stable. Over the next 12 hours, the hypoxia worsened, requiring intubation. A CBC showed a neutrophil count of 5200/$mm^3$, Hb of 10.5 g/dl, and platelet count of 90,000/$mm^3$. Coagulation studies revealed evidence of disseminated intravascular coagulation. ABG analysis on assist control mode at a rate of 14 breaths/min, tidal volume of 700 ml, $Fio_2$ of 0.5, and PEEP of 5 cm $H_2O$ showed a pH of 7.36, $Paco_2$ of 30 mm Hg, $Pao_2$ of 50 mm Hg, and oxygen saturation of 80%. Plateau airway pressure was measured at 28 cm $H_2O$. A CXR film revealed diffuse four-quadrant interstitial and alveolar infiltration.

The above measurements show the patient to have a static compliance of 30 ml/cm $H_2O$ and a lung injury score of 3, indicating severe lung injury.

Proper correction of hypoxia in this patient would entail increasing the level of $Fio_2$ to 100%. However, increasing the level of inspired oxygen to 60% is considered to increase lung damage from oxygen toxicity. Therefore PEEP should be increased in 2.5 to 5 cm increments until $Fio_2$ can be decreased to safe concentrations while maintaining $Pao_2$ >55 mm Hg. CO must be monitored because increasing levels of PEEP may adversely affect both CO and oxygen delivery. Inotropic support after adequate volume replacement can be used to maintain appropriate CO and oxygen delivery in these instances.

The mortality in patients such as the one described here approaches 90% in some studies. Alternative investigational methods of ventilation may be considered, such as inverse inspiratory/expiratory ratio ventilation or extracorporeal gas exchange, if conventional methods of ventilation are unsuccessful.

# CHAPTER 20

# *Life-Threatening Bronchospasm*

R. Phillip Dellinger

## CASE 1

A 48-year-old woman came to the hospital with severe abdominal pain. She had peritoneal signs and underwent laparotomy, during which a perforated appendix was diagnosed and treated. The patient's medical history included a 10-pack-year cigarette-smoking habit and childhood asthma. At the time, the patient was taking anhydrous theophylline 200 mg bid and using an albuterol inhaler prn. She admitted to being hospitalized twice in the past for what she was told was "bronchitis" and "asthma." She had not smoked in the last 5 years. She also stated that she had been prescribed steroid pills several times in the past for her breathing problem. The patient initially did well postoperatively and was extubated without difficulty. One day following extubation, she complained of shortness of breath. She was found to be tachypneic and had diffuse wheezes. Her current medication for bronchospasm was prn inhaler only.

- *What should your initial therapeutic decision be in this case?*

The medication of choice for acute bronchospasm is inhaled beta-2 selective agonists. Nebulization of albuterol or metaproterenol would be appropriate for this patient. The severity of the patient's bronchospasm and the risk for beta-1 side effects would dictate the frequency of inhalation therapy. This patient has minimal risks for beta-1 cardiac toxicity.

- *What is the role of subcutaneous beta-agonists in this case?*

In this patient with moderate acute symptoms, it would be most appropriate to begin treatment with inhaled beta-agonists, and, pending response, to withhold subcutaneous beta-agonists, which would be associated with greater chance of cardiac side effects.

- *Should this patient receive intravenous steroids?*

Since the overwhelming majority of patients with bronchospasm have underlying inflammation, as a general rule, anti-inflammatory therapy should be initiated. For the acutely bronchospastic patient, intravenous steroids are appropriate, and this patient has a history of steroid therapy. This patient should be given methylprednisolone 60 to 125 mg IV, with the dose repeated every 4 to 6 hours. As the patient improves, a conversion to oral steroid is appropriate.

- *What is the role of intravenous aminophylline in this case?*

---

This chapter can be studied in conjunction with *Essentials of Surgical Critical Care,* edited by Jerome H. Abrams and Frank B. Cerra (St. Louis: Quality Medical Publishing, Inc., 1993), Chapters 24, *26,* and 27. Italicized number indicates the main chapter reference.

The role of intravenous aminophylline in acute bronchospasm is questionable. Although some studies demonstrate a significant adjunctive response when this agent is added to inhaled beta-agonists, meta-analysis fails to show a significant benefit. Therefore the use of intravenous aminophylline in this patient is controversial. If intravenous aminophylline is used, it is important to consider coexisting toxic factors such as hypokalemia or coronary artery disease prior to administration. If the patient is not currently taking theophylline, then a loading dose of aminophylline, 6 mg/kg over 45 minutes, is appropriate, followed by maintenance doses.

- *What is the role of inhaled anticholinergics in this case?*

The use of anticholinergics such as ipratropium by metered-dose inhaler has better results when added to beta-agonist therapy than does intravenous aminophylline. The patient with mild or moderate symptoms who responds quickly to inhaled beta-agonists does not need anticholinergic therapy added. If this patient's bronchospasm worsened or failed to improve, anticholinergic therapy would be appropriate.

Albuterol inhalation therapy was initiated as well as methylprednisolone 125 mg IV. The patient's bronchospasm did not improve, and the patient appeared to be worse after 45 minutes of therapy.

- *At this point, what is the best measure of the patient's bronchospasm status?*

First, based on the patient's deteriorating condition, ipratropium should be added. The response from ipratropium would not be expected to be seen for at least 30 minutes. Judging the severity of bronchospasm is notoriously difficult. This patient's worsening signs of distress suggest a serious condition, but objective measurements are needed. Peak expiratory flow rate is found to be 120 L/min.

- *What would the estimated normal peak flow rate be for this patient, who is 5 feet, 5 inches tall?*

This 48-year-old woman would have an estimated peak flow rate of 450 L/min. Higher peak flow rates are found in younger patients (once adulthood is reached), in taller patients, and in men.

ABG analysis revealed a pH of 7.3, partial pressure of carbon dioxide ($Paco_2$) of 40 mm Hg, and partial pressure of oxygen ($Po_2$) of 160 mm Hg.

- *What is the interpretation of the ABG data?*

The ABG data reveal a normal $Paco_2$ with an acidotic pH. Most patients with acute bronchospasm hyperventilate and maintain a decreased $Paco_2$, which produces respiratory alkalosis. Patients with chronic (lasting several days) hyperventilation secondary to unremitting bronchospasm may have a chronic respiratory alkalosis with renal excretion of bicarbonate to normalize pH. Since this patient's bronchospasm was acute, this should not be the case. Therefore the acidosis in this patient must be assumed to be a primary disorder and raises the ominous possibility of lactate accumulation secondary to imminent diaphragm failure. In addition, normal or slightly elevated $Paco_2$ in a patient with significant distress implies that the patient is fatigued. The normal $Paco_2$ soon will be followed by a rise in $Paco_2$ and acute ventilatory failure. Therefore intubation of the patient should be considered at this time.

The patient was reintubated and placed on mechanical ventilator support.

- *What considerations are needed for determining the dosage of inhaled beta-agonists and ipratropium in this patient, who is now mechanically ventilated?*

Delivery of aerosol medications in the intubated patient is associated with significant deposition on the endotracheal tube, which produces a significant reduction in the effective dose. Therefore doubling the dosage for the intubated patient should be considered.

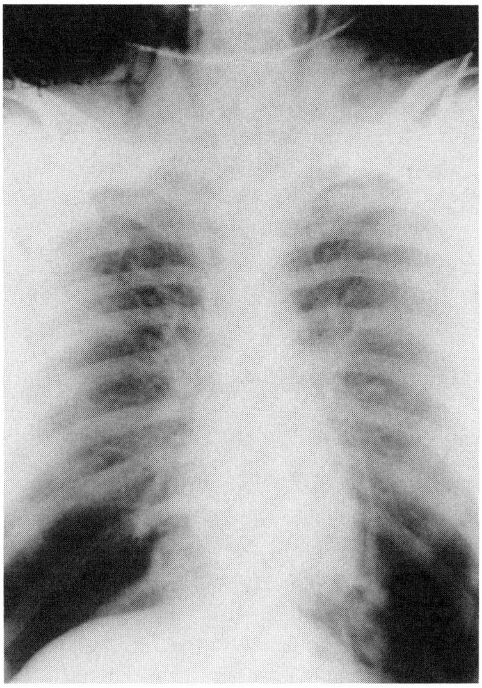

FIG 20-1

## CASE 2

As the surgical resident on call for consultation, you were called to the ICU to evaluate a 32-year-old patient who was admitted to the unit 3 hours earlier for status asthmaticus. She was receiving albuterol q 1 hr, ipratropium by metered-dose inhaler and spacer q 6 hr, and intravenous methylprednisolone 125 mg q 4 hr (intravenous aminophylline had not been instituted). You were asked to review the CXR film, which was diagnosed by the medicine housestaff as demonstrating pneumomediastinum. The concern was whether chest tube insertion was indicated. Before you were able to review the film, the physicians were called to the bedside because the patient was "in extremis." The patient was intubated and placed on mechanical ventilator support. A repeat CXR film was obtained. While the second film was being processed, the patient became severely hypotensive. The initial CXR film you were called to evaluate is shown in Fig. 20-1.

- *Based on this film, what is the likely reason for the patient's hypotension? What are other potential reasons for hypotension unrelated to the CXR?*

The patient's CXR film demonstrates pneumomediastinum and subcutaneous air. The radiolucent areas overlying the diaphragm are compatible with bilateral pneumothorax. In this patient, who became hypotensive following intubation, tension pneumothorax should be considered. Auscultation of the patient's chest revealed minimal air movement on either side. The chest was bilaterally tympanitic.

- *Consideration for the patient's diagnosis at this time includes which conditions?*

Although bilateral tension pneumothorax would be unusual, it is certainly possible in this patient. The decision to insert bilateral needle thoracostomies in this patient would be contro-

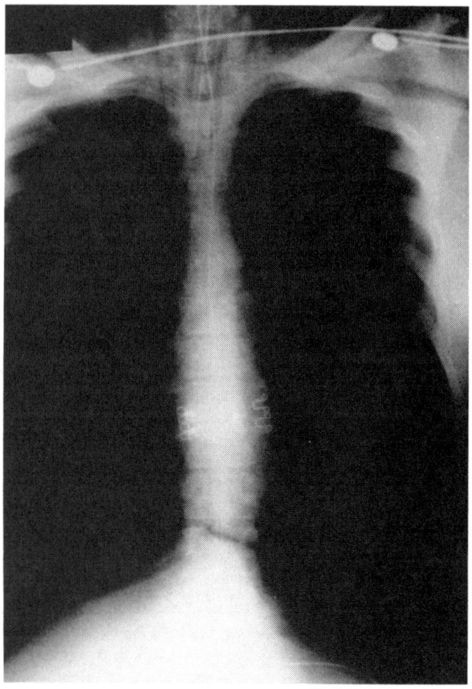

FIG 20-2

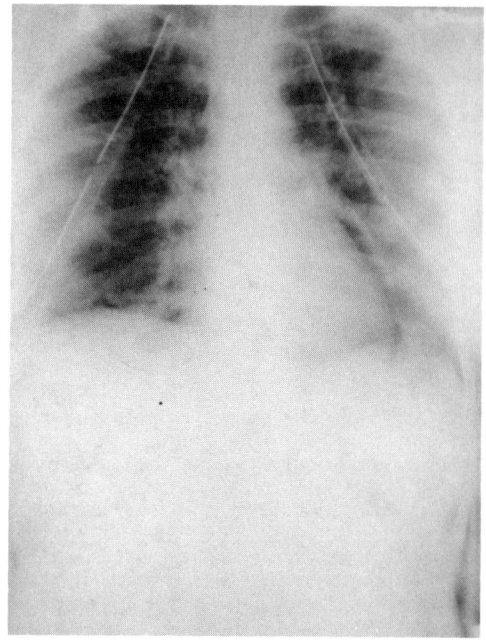

FIG 20-3

versial, but in the severely hypotensive patient it might be life-saving. The other possibility would be intrinsic positive end-expiratory pressure (PEEP) secondary to inadequate expiratory time from the high minute ventilation. This is particularly a problem if the assist control mode was selected and the patient was allowed to trigger larger inspired tidal volumes.

The repeat CXR film following intubation is shown in Fig. 20-2.

- *What is the diagnosis?*

This patient has bilateral tension pneumothorax with "vanishing heart" and "inverted diaphragm" on the left side. Bilateral needle thoracostomies were performed in the second intercostal space bilaterally, and chest tube placement followed. A repeat CXR film following chest tube placement is shown in Fig. 20-3. The patient's condition stabilized, but she continued to have severe wheezing and required high peak inspiratory pressures for mechanical ventilation. Despite high peak airway pressures, the patient's $PaCO_2$ remained elevated at 66 mm Hg with a pH of 7.18.

- *What other therapeutic considerations are relevant at this time?*

This patient did not respond to inhaled beta-agonist, inhaled anticholinergics, and intravenous steroids. The possibility is good that the patient will have a delayed response to anti-inflammatory medications. However, in the interim the patient required considerable ventilator support and high peak inspiratory pressures. High peak airway (inspiratory) pressures may result in high tidal volumes in areas of the lung less involved with the asthma inflammatory process. The use of iatrogenic alkalinization with bicarbonate would allow the pH to rise to a concentration more compatible with effective bronchodilator action (in patients with currently high $PaCO_2$ and low pH) or to achieve the capability to decrease minute ventilation and lower peak airway pressures to lessen the possibility of barotrauma (in patients with currently normal $PaCO_2$ and normal pH but high peak airway pressures).

# CHAPTER 21

# *Conventional Ventilator Support*

Karl L. Yang • Guillermo Gutierrez

## CASE 1

A 59-year-old man with a history of chronic obstructive pulmonary disease was admitted to the SICU in respiratory failure. The initial ABG analysis obtained in the emergency room showed pH of 7.15, partial pressure of oxygen ($Pao_2$) of 47 mm Hg, and partial pressure of carbon dioxide ($Paco_2$) of 78 mm Hg while the patient was breathing room air. He was intubated and started on assist control mode mechanical ventilation. The initial settings of the ventilator were respiratory rate 20 breaths/min, tidal volume 800 ml, and fraction of inspired oxygen ($Fio_2$) of 1. The patient made no spontaneous breathing effort. The ABG analysis obtained 30 minutes after the initiation of ventilatory support showed a pH of 7.56, $Pao_2$ of 358 mm Hg, and $Paco_2$ of 32 mm Hg. Blood pressure was 90/60 mm Hg. The respiratory rate was then reduced to 10 breaths/min, and subsequent ABG analysis revealed the resolution of the respiratory alkalosis. Despite the adequacy of mechanical ventilation, the patient continued to show mild respiratory distress and paradoxical breathing. Blood pressure remained about 100/60 mm Hg. The patient was noted to have an intrinsic positive end-expiratory pressure (PEEP) of 11 cm $H_2O$. At this time, 8 cm $H_2O$ of PEEP was added, and fluid resuscitation was started. Soon thereafter, the paradoxical breathing and hypotension resolved.

This case illustrates several salient features of the problems that improper ventilator settings can create for the patient.

This patient developed severe respiratory alkalosis because the initial respiratory rate was too high. Instead of routinely setting a high ventilator rate, the rate should be adjusted until the patient begins to trigger the ventilator spontaneously. This observation is especially important in patients with chronic obstructive pulmonary disease (COPD) who already may have a compensated respiratory acidosis. With the sudden imposition of respiratory alkalosis, the kidneys will begin to excrete bicarbonate. As a result of this loss of bicarbonate, the weaning process becomes much more difficult since the patient will need to increase the minute ventilation in order to maintain an adequate pH.

Despite the adequacy of the ABG concentrations while he was being ventilated, this patient continued to have paradoxical breathing. This finding should alert the physician to look for the presence of intrinsic PEEP. Intrinsic PEEP occurs when there is inadequate time for expiration.

This chapter can be studied in conjunction with *Essentials of Surgical Critical Care,* edited by Jerome H. Abrams and Frank B. Cerra (St. Louis: Quality Medical Publishing, Inc., 1993), Chapters 24, 25, *27,* 28, and 54. Italicized number indicates the main chapter reference.

Intrinsic PEEP is frequently encountered in COPD patients because prolonged expiratory time is needed to exhale tidal volume completely. In order to trigger the ventilator, the patient needs to generate a subatmospheric, or negative, pressure equal to the sum of the trigger sensitivity and the intrinsic PEEP. This problem can be minimized by simply adding external PEEP. The relatively large tidal volume used in this case also can increase the likelihood of intrinsic PEEP. As long as external PEEP is lower than the intrinsic PEEP, there should not be hemodynamic alterations. In this patient the addition of external PEEP helped to eliminate paradoxical breathing without decreasing cardiac output.

## CASE 2

A 23-year-old woman was intubated because of respiratory distress. A CXR film revealed diffuse interstitial infiltrates. The patient had a history of Hodgkin's lymphoma treated with doxorubicin, bleomycin, vinblastin, and dacarbazine. She had received her last chemotherapy treatment approximately 10 days earlier. She had severe pancytopenia, and the $Pa{O_2}$ was 63 mm Hg on $FI{O_2}$ of 1. At this point, 5 cm $H_2O$ of PEEP was added to improve the arterial oxygen concentration. Eventually PEEP was increased to 17 cm $H_2O$ in order to maintain a $Pa{O_2}$ of 76 mm Hg. At this level of PEEP, the patient's blood pressure decreased to 85/40 mm Hg and a pulmonary artery catheter was placed to monitor hemodynamics. The pulmonary artery pressure was 36/19 mm Hg, and the pulmonary artery occlusion pressure (PAOP) was 12 mm Hg. The patient was given fluids and RBC transfusions, resulting in significant hemodynamic improvement.

This is a case of adult respiratory distress syndrome (ARDS), probably resulting from sepsis. PEEP ventilation is frequently utilized in ARDS to improve oxygenation and to lower $FI{O_2}$ requirements. The risk of oxygen toxicity in this particular patient was substantial because she had previously received bleomycin, which can synergistically act with oxygen to increase oxygen toxicity to the lung. Thus vigorous attempts to lower $FI{O_2}$ were warranted. With the addition of PEEP, this patient developed hypotension even though her PAOP seemed adequate. It is important to realize that PAOP is often elevated during PEEP ventilation, while the left ventricular filling volume may be relatively low. This phenomenon occurs because of the transmission of airway pressure to the pericardial surface. Increased airway pressure is caused by hyperinflation of the lung. Thus PAOP of 12 mm Hg is not an adequate filling pressure if the patient is receiving PEEP of 15 cm $H_2O$. In order to overcome the effect of PEEP, fluid resuscitation is the most frequently used therapy. In this patient the selection of RBC transfusion was most appropriate since it not only corrected the volume status but also improved the oxygen delivery to the peripheral tissues.

# CHAPTER 22

## *Strategies for Pulmonary Support When Conventional Ventilation Methods Fail*

Jerome H. Abrams

## CASE

A 24-year-old man was injured in a motor vehicle accident. The patient was the driver and was not wearing a seat belt at the time of his collision with a concrete embankment. His estimated speed was 45 miles per hour. The patient sustained the following injuries: bilateral pulmonary contusion, liver laceration, colon laceration, a pelvic fracture, and a left femur fracture. He was intubated shortly after arrival at the referring hospital. With a positive diagnostic peritoneal lavage, exploration was begun. The liver laceration was not bleeding at the time of exploration. The colon laceration was on the right side of the colon and was 1 cm in length. The referring surgeon performed a primary repair. The left femur fracture was internally fixed. The pelvic fracture was stable. After the injuries were stabilized, the patient made satisfactory clinical progress until hospital day 2. At that time the CXR film revealed diffuse bilateral alveolar infiltrates. The $Pa_{O_2}$ was 62 mm Hg while on $FI_{O_2}$ of 0.5. Over the next several hours, pulmonary function worsened and the patient required increased ventilator support. On hospital day 3, the patient was receiving an $FI_{O_2}$ of 0.9. Ventilator settings and arterial blood gas measurements were as follows:

| Mode | TV | RR | PEEP | $FI_{O_2}$ | $Sa_{O_2}$ | I:E | PAP | MAP | $Pa_{O_2}$ | $Pa_{CO_2}$ | pH | $HCO_3^-$ |
|---|---|---|---|---|---|---|---|---|---|---|---|---|
| AC | 950 | 16 | 8 | 0.9 | 89 | 1:3 | 46 | 19 | 58 | 36 | 7.43 | 23 |

- *Would you change the ventilator management of this patient?*

Despite a significantly elevated $FI_{O_2}$, the patient demonstrates a low $Pa_{O_2}$ with marginal arterial oxygen saturation. At this point in his clinical course, he demonstrates satisfactory alveolar ventilation. The acute lung injury is of recent onset. Elevated $FI_{O_2}$ probably exacerbates lung injury. In my judgment, elevated $FI_{O_2}$ represents greater toxicity to the cellular components of the alveoli than does a moderate increase in mean airway pressure. Since mean airway pressure is well below 30 cm $H_2O$, an increase in PEEP is ordered.

The PEEP is increased in increments of 2 cm $H_2O$ from 8 to 14 cm $H_2O$. The ventilator settings and arterial blood gas measurements obtained on these settings were:

| Mode | TV | RR | PEEP | $FI_{O_2}$ | $Sa_{O_2}$ | I:E | PAP | MAP | $Pa_{O_2}$ | $Pa_{CO_2}$ | pH | $HCO_3^-$ |
|---|---|---|---|---|---|---|---|---|---|---|---|---|
| AC | 950 | 16 | 14 | 0.5 | 96 | 1:3 | 49 | 23 | 83 | 39 | 7.39 | 22 |

This chapter can be studied in conjunction with *Essentials of Surgical Critical Care,* edited by Jerome H. Abrams and Frank B. Cerra (St. Louis: Quality Medical Publishing, Inc., 1993), Chapters 5, 11, 25, 27, *28,* and 54. Italicized number indicates the main chapter reference.

▪ *What is your analysis of the patient's pulmonary support at this time?*

Increasing the PEEP from 8 to 14 cm $H_2O$ has resulted in an increase in mean airway pressure and a smaller change in peak airway pressure. With these maneuvers, the $FIO_2$ has been lowered, and the patient's arterial oxygen saturation has increased. Although increasing PEEP usually will increase $PaCO_2$ ($\uparrow V_D/V_T$) for constant respiratory rate, at this time clearance of carbon dioxide is satisfactory.

The patient improved until hospital day 5, when evidence of tension pneumothorax appeared. Tube thoracostomy was performed, and the lung was shown as reexpanded on the CXR film following chest tube placement. The patient demonstrated a small but continuous air leak.

▪ *What is your approach to the patient at this time?*

The patient now has acute lung injury of somewhat greater than 5 days' duration. Efforts at maintaining functional residual capacity with the use of PEEP have resulted in evidence of barotrauma. Experimental lung injury demonstrates injury to type I pneumocytes in acute lung injury of less than 5 days' duration. By the fifth day after injury, alveoli are populated by type II pneumocytes, and large areas of denuded basement membrane are observed. Patients who are managed with extracorporeal support have demonstrated lung repair, despite being maintained on $FIO_2$ of 1. At this point in the patient's clinical course, my judgment is that elevated airway pressures represent a greater potential for injury than do other components of his ventilator management. With such noncompliant lungs, additional strategies for maintaining oxygenation require distribution of oxygen-containing gas to alveoli that maintain communication with the tracheobronchial tree. The appearance of a significant air leak could seriously compromise oxygenation by providing a low-resistance pathway for oxygenated inspired gas to escape.

After the PEEP was reduced from 14 to 10 cm $H_2O$ and the tidal volume was reduced by 10%, ventilator settings and arterial blood gas determinations were as follows:

| Mode | TV | RR | PEEP | $FIO_2$ | $SaO_2$ | I:E | PAP | MAP | $PaO_2$ | $PaCO_2$ | pH | $HCO_3^-$ |
|---|---|---|---|---|---|---|---|---|---|---|---|---|
| AC | 850 | 16 | 10 | 0.5 | 95 | 1:3 | 39 | 20 | 72 | 41 | 7.39 | 24 |

▪ *What is your approach to a patient with these findings?*

Both reducing the PEEP and decreasing the tidal volume have decreased the airway pressures somewhat. The patient continues to have an air leak, and efforts to reduce the pressures further may help prevent additional barotrauma and reduce the air leak. Accordingly, the tidal volume is reduced further. It is reduced gradually, by decrements of 10%, until it measures 600 ml. To maintain comparable alveolar ventilation, the respiratory rate is increased with each decrement of tidal volume. With a tidal volume of 600 ml, the following arterial blood gas measurements are obtained at the ventilator settings shown:

| Mode | TV | RR | PEEP | $FIO_2$ | $SaO_2$ | I:E | PAP | MAP | $PaO_2$ | $PaCO_2$ | pH | $HCO_3^-$ |
|---|---|---|---|---|---|---|---|---|---|---|---|---|
| AC | 600 | 24 | 10 | 0.8 | 84 | 1:2 | 40 | 18 | 58 | 46 | 7.36 | 25 |

▪ *What is your approach to the patient's ventilator management?*

Reducing the tidal volume has satisfactorily decreased airway pressures to the target values of peak airway pressure <45 and mean airway pressure <30. The consequence of reducing airway pressure is worsening arterial oxygen saturation. Presumably, the inspired breath is not being distributed to all alveoli that are exchanging gas. The $FIO_2$ is again high. Since the patient's acute lung injury is now of several days' duration, my judgment is that increased airway pressures continue to represent a greater risk to the patient at this point in his clinical course than does an elevated $FIO_2$. Despite the elevated $FIO_2$, the arterial oxygen saturation is marginal. Presumably, damaged airways are present that have extremely long time constants, compared to others, for exchange of gas. For this reason, holding inspiration longer may allow the inspired gas flow to distribute itself more effectively. At this point, the I:E ratio is increased.

With the aid of the attending intensivist, the I:E ratio was gradually increased from 1:2 to 2:1. Prior to inverting the I:E ratio, the patient was sedated and paralyzed. The following arterial blood gas measurements were obtained at the ventilator settings indicated:

| Mode | TV | RR | PEEP | $FIO_2$ | $SaO_2$ | I:E | PAP | MAP | $PaO_2$ | $PaCO_2$ | pH | $HCO_3^-$ |
|---|---|---|---|---|---|---|---|---|---|---|---|---|
| PC-IRV | 600 | 24 | 10 | 0.8 | 91 | 2:1 | 40 | 20 | 70 | 62 | 7.29 | 26 |

- *What is your evaluation of the patient at this time?*

Inverting the I:E ratio had succeeded in increasing the arterial oxygen saturation. This maneuver, while successful in improving oxygenation, has compromised alveolar ventilation and has produced increasing respiratory acidosis.

Renal mechanisms are expected to allow the patient to significantly compensate his acidemia over the next 36 to 48 hours. With airway pressures below the maximum clinical target and satisfactory $SaO_2$, the present conditions are continued.

Over the following 36 hours, the patient's renal function deteriorated. He became oliguric and produced only 400 ml of urine for 24 hours. In addition, pulmonary compliance and pulmonary hypertension also worsened. Tidal volume was decreased in stepwise fashion and the respiratory rate was increased. Repeat arterial blood gas measurements on the following ventilator settings were noted:

| Mode | TV | RR | PEEP | $FIO_2$ | $SaO_2$ | I:E | PAP | MAP | $PaO_2$ | $PaCO_2$ | pH | $HCO_3^-$ |
|---|---|---|---|---|---|---|---|---|---|---|---|---|
| PC-IRV | 450 | 42 | 12 | 0.8 | 88 | 2.5:1 | 44 | 22 | 68 | 63 | 7.11 | 18 |

- *What is your approach to the patient at this time?*

A tragic situation has developed. A young patient with isolated pulmonary failure has reached the limits of conventional pulmonary support. Although he is able to oxygenate his blood with his native lungs, he is unable to eliminate carbon dioxide. His acidosis is now combined respiratory and metabolic acidosis. With the demonstrated failure of conventional ventilation, the ability to oxygenate blood with native lungs, and the failure to excrete carbon dioxide, extracorporeal carbon dioxide removal (ECCOR) is one of the few therapies remaining.

You must continue to search for a septic focus and be certain not to provide excess calories or carbohydrates to prevent excess production of carbon dioxide. Since your hospital is experienced with ECCOR, you institute ECCOR therapy.

Femoral and internal jugular catheters were placed percutaneously. ECCOR was begun without incident. After the patient's condition became stabilized on ECCOR, arterial oxygen saturation, elimination of carbon dioxide, and pulmonary artery pressures all improved. The patient remained on extracorporeal support for 1 week and was successfully weaned from this support. He was then weaned from conventional ventilation over 2 weeks. The patient was discharged to home and outpatient rehabilitation was continued.

SECTION 4 *Renal Function*

# CHAPTER 23

# *Disturbances of Acid-Base Homeostasis*

Jon F. Berlauk

## CASE 1

A 48-year-old man was transferred from a hospital ward to the SICU because of severe respiratory distress. His nurse reported that the patient was recovering uneventfully from a femoropopliteal bypass operation 8 days before and expected to be discharged the next morning. She had left him with his dinner only 15 minutes prior to this "asthma attack." The patient's medical history included long-standing diabetes mellitus complicated by renal insufficiency, severe peripheral vascular disease, and a myocardial infarction six months earlier. He had not received medications since late morning.

Examination revealed a confused, dyspneic man unable to talk. Auscultation of the chest revealed bilateral inspiratory and expiratory wheezes and rhonchi.

*Vital signs*

| BP | P | RR | Temp |
|---|---|---|---|
| 180/100 | 132 | 20 | 98.6° F |

Laboratory analyses gave the following values:

*ABG on $F_{IO_2}$ = 0.21*

| pH | $P_{CO_2}$ | $P_{O_2}$ | $HCO_3^-$ |
|---|---|---|---|
| 7.18 | 80 | 56 | 28 |

*Electrolytes*

| Na | K | Cl | $HCO_3^-$ |
|---|---|---|---|
| 140 | 5 | 100 | 30 |

- *What is your evaluation?*

This chapter can be studied in conjunction with *Essentials of Surgical Critical Care,* edited by Jerome H. Abrams and Frank B. Cerra (St. Louis: Quality Medical Publishing, Inc., 1993), Chapter 29.

The differential diagnosis should include pulmonary embolism (PE), gastric aspiration, foreign body aspiration, allergic reaction (severe bronchospasm), and myocardial infarction (MI).

## ACID-BASE ANALYSIS*

Step 1: The patient has severe acidosis.

Step 2: The calculated pH = 7.2 based on the assumption that the partial pressure of carbon dioxide ($Pco_2$) abruptly increased to 80 mm Hg and is responsible for the pH measured on ABG analysis.

Step 3: There is good correlation between measured and calculated pH; therefore the diagnosis of acute respiratory acidosis can be made.

Step 4: To confirm this diagnosis, verify that the $HCO_3^-$ increased ~ 1 mEq/L for each 10 mm Hg increase in $Pco_2$ (Henderson-Hasselbalch re-equilibration). For an acute 40 mm Hg increase in $Pco_2$, you would expect an increase in $HCO_3^-$ ~ 4 mEq/L or $HCO_3^-$ to equal 28 mEq/L on ABG analysis. The diagnosis is confirmed.

Anion gap (AG): 140 − (100 + 30) = 10 mEq/L, a normal value.

■ ■ ■

Based on the ABG analysis and available clinical data, neither MI, allergic reaction, nor massive PE is likely. Bronchoscopy revealed a piece of meat lodged in the trachea. This patient had acute respiratory acidosis secondary to foreign body aspiration.

**BIBLIOGRAPHY**

Kilburn KH. Neurologic manifestations of respiratory failure. Arch Intern Med 116:409, 1965.

## CASE 2

The code blue team was paged to a general surgical ward during an evening when you were covering the SICU. Thirty minutes later the SICU charge nurse handed you a slip of paper and announced, "We have an emergency admission from general surgery. This is all I know about the patient." Printed on the paper was the following:

STAT LABS 7:10 PM

*ABG on $Fio_2$ = 1*

| pH | $Pco_2$ | $Po_2$ | $HCO_3^-$ |
|---|---|---|---|
| 7.1 | 70 | 35 | 20.5 |

- *What is your interpretation of these data?*

## ACID-BASE ANALYSIS

Step 1: The patient has severe acidosis.

Step 2: The calculated pH = 7.25.

---

*The SICU physician can rely on fairly simple and practical guidelines to interpret ABG data. Four steps are involved:

1. Check the pH.
2. Assume all perturbations in pH are due to an *acute* change in $Pco_2$.
3. Confirm or refute this assumption (diagnose the primary acid-base disorder).
4. Check for normal physiologic compensation (diagnose the secondary acid-base disorder, if present).

Step 3: Calculated and measured pH are both acidotic; therefore the patient has respiratory acidosis. However, the calculated pH did not predict the measured pH. Since the measured pH is more acidotic than the calculated pH, you should diagnose combined respiratory acidosis and metabolic acidosis. (There is only one *mixed* disorder that cannot be differentiated from a combined disorder by ABG analysis alone. See Case 7). It is tempting to infer from this analysis that the respiratory acidosis was the primary disorder and metabolic acidosis was secondary, but do not fall into the trap. A single ABG analysis of a complex acid-base disorder does not provide such specific information.

Step 4: This step is not helpful in analyzing this ABG. By definition, there is no compensation with a combined disorder.

Even with the limited information available, you can form a preliminary differential diagnosis of a sudden event resulting in cardiac and pulmonary failure: massive PE, cardiac arrest, massive air embolism, and anaphylaxis.

This patient was a 56-year-old man hospitalized earlier in the day with upper abdominal pain. He was transferred to the SICU.

Examination revealed an unresponsive, intubated patient who was being mechanically ventilated.

*Vital signs*

| BP | P | RR | Temp |
|---|---|---|---|
| 88/60 | 106 | 12 | 99° F |

Laboratory studies gave the following values:

*ABG on $FIO_2$ = 0.4*

| pH | $PCO_2$ | $PO_2$ | $HCO_3^-$ |
|---|---|---|---|
| 7.3 | 38 | 87 | 17 |

*Electrolytes*

| Na | K | Cl | $HCO_3^-$ |
|---|---|---|---|
| 139 | 4.4 | 95 | 22 |

- *What is the patient's acid-base disorder?*

## ACID-BASE ANALYSIS

Step 1: The patient still has mild acidosis.

Step 2: The calculated pH = 7.44.

Step 3: Calculated and measured pH now lie in opposite directions of pH = 7.4; therefore the acidosis is metabolic. The bicarbonate now reflects the primary disorder, and compensation (if any) should be respiratory.

Step 4: Winter's formula (simplified): 1.5 (17) + 8 ± 2 = 35.5 for the highest $PCO_2$ expected. In addition, the last two digits of the pH (i.e., 30) do not correlate well with the measured $PCO_2$ (i.e., 38). A secondary disorder is present, that is, respiratory acidosis (iatrogenic?).

AG = 139 − (95 + 22) = 22. The most likely diagnosis for the increased AG acidosis is lactic acidosis from poor tissue perfusion.

Appropriate adjustments were made on the ventilator. An ECG revealed a large inferior MI, which was treated appropriately. This patient had a combined acid-base disorder of respiratory acidosis and metabolic acidosis secondary to cardiac arrest.

## CASE 3

After you stabilized the condition of the patient in Case 2, you were asked to attend to his wife in the family waiting room. She was reported to have "nearly fainted" and then complained of difficulty "catching her breath" and "tightness" in her chest. She gave a history of "heart palpitations" but had no other medical problems.

Examination revealed an overweight, anxious, middle-aged woman lying on a couch and clutching her chest.

*Vital signs*

| BP | P | RR | Temp |
|---|---|---|---|
| 146/98 | 126 | 28 | 98.8° F |

You administer nasal oxygen, order an ECG, and send a blood sample for an ABG analysis.

*ECG: Sinus tachycardia; nonspecific ST-T segment changes in the lateral precordial leads.*

*ABG on 2 L nasal $O_2$*

| pH | $PCO_2$ | $PO_2$ | $HCO_3^-$ |
|---|---|---|---|
| 7.6 | 20 | 141 | 20 |

- *What is your evaluation?*

Your differential diagnosis should include cardiac dysrhythmia, MI, cerebrovascular accident, hypoglycemia, allergic reaction, and hyperventilation syndrome.

## ACID-BASE ANALYSIS

Step 1: The patient has severe alkalosis.
Step 2: The calculated pH = 7.6.
Step 3: Calculated and measured pH correlate exactly. The patient has acute respiratory alkalosis.
Step 4: To confirm this interpretation, the $HCO_3^-$ would be expected to decrease ~ 5 mEq for an acute 20 mm Hg decrease in $PCO_2$. You expect the $HCO_3^-$ ~ 19 mEq/L, and it is the same, within error, as the measured value.

The patient felt much better after breathing into a paper bag for several minutes. She admitted to feeling frightened and helpless because of her husband's serious condition. Your reassurance worked wonders. This woman had acute respiratory alkalosis secondary to anxiety-provoked hyperventilation.

### BIBLIOGRAPHY

Lary D, Goldschlager N. Electrocardiographic changes during hyperventilation in patients with normal coronary arteriograms. Am Heart J 87:383, 1974.

Margarian GJ. Hyperventilation syndromes: Infrequently recognized common expressions of anxiety and stress. Medicine 61:219, 1982.

Saltzman H, Heyman A, Sieker H. Correlation of clinical and physiological manifestation of sustained hyperventilation. N Engl J Med 268:1431, 1963.

## CASE 4

An 81-year-old man with chronic emphysema and severe peripheral vascular disease was sent to the hospital from his nursing home with a "cold leg." He was evaluated in the emergency department and scheduled for an emergency operation to remove a suspected arterial occlusion. The patient was recovering in the postanesthesia recovery room when you received a call from the surgery resident, who informed you that the patient did well intraoperatively but then failed several attempts at being weaned from the ventilator. The resident wanted to admit the patient to the SICU. He was unable to interpret the latest ABG data.

*ABG on* $F_{IO_2} = 0.4$

| pH | $P_{CO_2}$ | $P_{O_2}$ | $HCO_3^-$ |
|---|---|---|---|
| 7.59 | 42 | 109 | 40 |

- *What is your evaluation of this acid-base disorder? Does this ABG analysis make sense?*

### ACID-BASE ANALYSIS

Step 1: The patient has severe alkalosis.
Step 2: The calculated pH = 7.39.
Step 3: Calculated and measured pH are on opposite sides of pH = 7.4; therefore the patient has metabolic alkalosis.
Step 4: You expect the $P_{CO_2}$ to rise ~ 6 mm Hg for each 10 mEq increase in $HCO_3^-$, or an expected $P_{CO_2}$ ~ 49 mm Hg. Since the measured $P_{CO_2}$ is lower, this patient also has respiratory alkalosis (probably iatrogenic).

The patient appears to have combined metabolic and respiratory alkalosis. From the limited clinical information given, you would have expected chronic respiratory acidosis if the patient had severe chronic obstructive pulmonary disease. You even may have anticipated metabolic acidosis if the patient had poor perfusion to his leg. It seems difficult to explain an alkalosis. Should you order a urinary chloride test?

You went to the postanesthesia recovery room to evaluate the situation. The nursing home records showed baseline laboratory studies:

*ABG on 1 L nasal* $O_2$

| pH | $P_{CO_2}$ | $P_{O_2}$ | $HCO_3^-$ |
|---|---|---|---|
| 7.31 | 75 | 58 | 37 |

*Electrolytes*

| Na | K | Cl | $HCO_3^-$ |
|---|---|---|---|
| 136 | 3.7 | 84 | 37 |

- *Do these data help you interpret the original ABG data?*

### ACID-BASE ANALYSIS

Step 1: The patient has acidosis.
Step 2: Calculated pH = 7.23.
Step 3: Diagnose respiratory acidosis.
Step 4: Compensation for a chronic 35 mm Hg elevation of $P_{CO_2}$ is about 12.2 mEq/L $HCO_3^-$ or an expected $HCO_3^-$ equal to 36.2 mEq/L on ABG analysis. The measured $HCO_3^-$ is 37 mEq/L; this ABG analysis shows chronic respiratory acidosis.

This patient has chronic respiratory acidosis because of his emphysema. His ventilation during the emergency operation was inappropriate for this pathophysiology. His $P_{CO_2}$ can decrease acutely, but the metabolic compensation ($\Delta$ $HCO_3^-$) cannot; therefore he appeared to have metabolic alkalosis. The patient's apneic threshold was much higher than normal, a result of his chronic emphysema. Attempts to wean him from the ventilator resulted in prolonged apnea. The patient has hypochloremia because of the compensation for chronic respiratory acidosis. If you measure urinary chloride, it should be low (<15 mEq/L).

■ ■ ■

This patient had posthypercapnic metabolic alkalosis and respiratory alkalosis from mechanical ventilation.

**BIBLIOGRAPHY**

Bear R, Goldstein M, Phillipson E, et al. Effect of metabolic alkalosis on respiratory function in patients with chronic obstructive lung disease. Can Med Assoc J 117:900, 1977.

Schwartz WB, Hays RM, Polak A, et al. Effects of chronic hypercapnia on electrolyte and acid-base equilibrium. II. Recovery, with special reference to the influence of chloride intake. J Clin Invest 40:1238, 1961.

## CASE 5

A frail 72-year-old man was admitted directly to the SICU from a nursing home. He was described as having "pneumonia." The patient had a history of chronic obstructive pulmonary disease and carcinoma of the lung. Eighteen months earlier he had a "lung resection" for the cancer and had been on continuous oxygen since that operation.

Examination revealed the patient to be cachectic, very lethargic, and cyanotic, with his breathing supported by nasal oxygen. He had a left thoracic surgical scar. Auscultation of the chest revealed poor breath sounds in all fields, but none at the right base.

*Vital signs*

| BP | P | RR | Temp |
|---|---|---|---|
| 90/62 | 144 | 30 | 103.6° F |

Laboratory analysis showed the following values:

*ABG on 2 L nasal $O_2$*

| pH | $Pco_2$ | $Po_2$ | $HCO_3^-$ |
|---|---|---|---|
| 7.22 | 85 | 50 | 34 |

■ *What is your evaluation? What should be done?*

## ACID-BASE ANALYSIS

Step 1: The patient has serious acidosis.

Step 2: The calculated pH = 7.18.

Step 3: Calculated and measured pH are both acidotic; therefore this patient has respiratory acidosis.

Step 4: The expected compensation for an acute 45 mm Hg increase in $Pco_2$ would be about 4.5 mEq/L $HCO_3^-$ or $HCO_3^-$ ~ 30 mEq/L. The expected compensation for a chronic 45 mm Hg increase in $Pco_2$ would be about 15.7 mEq/L $HCO_3^-$ or $HCO_3^-$ ~ 40 mEq/L. This patient has a measured bicarbonate between these two values.

Two explanations are possible: (1) the patient is still compensating for a severe episode of respiratory acidosis less than 36 hours ago, or (2) he has acute respiratory acidosis superimposed on chronic respiratory acidosis. The latter explanation seems more likely and can be confirmed with a baseline ABG analysis.

The difference between these interpretations is not trivial. There is little question that this patient requires intubation and assisted ventilation. However, if the first explanation is chosen, he will be inappropriately hyperventilated (see Case 4).

The patient was intubated and placed on mechanical ventilation to achieve an ABG analysis: 7.30/60/88/29. A baseline ABG analysis was obtained from his old records: 7.33/60/52/31. This patient had acute respiratory acidosis superimposed on chronic respiratory acidosis secondary to pneumonia in a setting of chronic respiratory failure.

**BIBLIOGRAPHY**

Kilburn KH. Shock, seizures, and coma with alkalosis during mechanical ventilation. Ann Intern Med 65:977, 1966.

## CASE 6

You were asked to see a 33-year-old woman in the emergency department. The emergency department resident did not know whether the patient needed to be admitted to the SICU and wanted your advice. The patient had a total colectomy 3 months earlier for ulcerative colitis. Her husband brought her to the emergency department because he suspected that she took an overdose of pills. He stated that she had been very depressed since her operation.

Examination revealed a thin, defiant woman who denied any problem.

*Vital signs*

| BP | P | RR | Temp |
|---|---|---|---|
| 110/82 | 128 | 30 | 100.2° F |

Laboratory studies gave the following values:

*ABG on $F_{IO_2}$ = 0.4*

| pH | $P_{CO_2}$ | $P_{O_2}$ | $HCO_3^-$ |
|---|---|---|---|
| 7.39 | 18 | 103 | 11 |

*Electrolytes*

| Na | K | Cl | $HCO_3^-$ |
|---|---|---|---|
| 138 | 3.9 | 99 | 11 |

- *What is your evaluation?*

## ACID-BASE ANALYSIS

Step 1: The pH is normal.

Step 2: The calculated pH = 7.62.

Step 3: With a normal pH and low $P_{CO_2}$, you should entertain the diagnosis of chronic respiratory alkalosis until the diagnosis is proven otherwise.

Step 4: Normal compensation for a chronic 22 mm Hg decrease in $P_{CO_2}$ is a decrease in $HCO_3^-$ ~ 11 mEq/L. This should give a measured $HCO_3^-$ ~ 13 mEq/L. The patient's $HCO_3^-$ is 11 mEq, which is outside the normal limits of compensation for chronic respiratory alkalosis. The patient has an additional metabolic disorder.

On calculation, the patient's AG = 27! Several toxins in the differential diagnosis of increased AG acidoses could cause an acidosis, but only one results in the mixed disorder of respiratory alkalosis and metabolic acidosis: salicylate intoxication.

After being confronted with the laboratory studies, the patient tearfully accepted admission to the SICU, where she was treated for salicylate overdose.

**BIBLIOGRAPHY**

Gabow PA, Anderson RJ, Potts DE, et al. Acid-base disturbances in the salicylate-intoxicated adult. Arch Intern Med 138:1481, 1978.

## CASE 7

The emergency department physician called to inform you of an SICU admission. A 62-year-old man with a history of diabetes mellitus, chronic obstructive pulmonary disease, and carcinoma of the larynx had respiratory failure. The patient had a radical neck dissection 6 months earlier for treatment of laryngeal cancer. Since that operation, he had several "asthma" attacks of increasing severity. He was in the emergency department 2 weeks earlier to receive epinephrine after inhaler medications failed to resolve an episode of severe bronchospasm. The patient developed another episode the previous morning and finally came to the emergency department at about noon that day. He had been in the emergency department for at least 6 hours, and intramuscular epinephrine (administered three times), intravenous aminophylline, and steroids had failed to reverse the patient's bronchospasm. His otolaryngology surgeon had examined him and did not believe that he had recurrent tumor, but bronchoscopy would be needed to make such a determination. The surgeon was about to perform the bronchoscopy when this ABG analysis was returned.

*ABG on* $F_{IO_2}$ *= 0.4*

| pH | $P_{CO_2}$ | $P_{O_2}$ | $HCO_3^-$ |
|---|---|---|---|
| 7.21 | 52 | 65 | 19 |

At this point the surgeon was worried about diabetic ketoacidosis or some kind of lactic acidosis. He wanted the patient admitted.

- *What is your evaluation?*

### ACID-BASE ANALYSIS

Step 1: This patient has significant acidosis.
Step 2: The calculated pH = 7.34.
Step 3: Since both calculated and measured pH are acidotic, this patient has respiratory acidosis. The measured pH is more acidotic than the calculated pH; therefore this ABG analysis shows combined respiratory and metabolic acidosis.
Step 4: This step is not helpful. The $HCO_3^-$ shows no compensation for a respiratory acidosis and is in fact low rather than elevated.

On the way to the emergency department you considered various combinations of causes for respiratory and metabolic acidosis: asthma and ketoacidosis, asthma and lactic acidosis, asthma and drug overdose, recurrent cancer and the above causes of metabolic acidosis.

In the emergency department, examination revealed a tired, dyspneic man leaning over several pillows. Chest auscultation showed diffuse bilateral expiratory wheezes. Decreased sounds were noted at both lung bases. Stridor was not noted.

*Vital signs*

| BP | P | RR | Temp |
|---|---|---|---|
| 170/110 | 132 | 28 | 98.4° F |

Laboratory studies gave the following values:

*ABG on $F_{IO_2}$ = 0.4*

| pH | $P_{CO_2}$ | $P_{O_2}$ | $HCO_3^-$ |
|---|---|---|---|
| 7.21 | 52 | 65 | 19 |

*Electrolytes*

| Na | K | Cl | $HCO_3^-$ |
|---|---|---|---|
| 142 | 3.5 | 112 | 20 |

Fingerstick glucose ~ 160 mg%.

In addition, an earlier ABG analysis at 12:32 PM revealed:

*ABG on $F_{IO_2}$ = 0.21*

| pH | $P_{CO_2}$ | $P_{O_2}$ | $HCO_3^-$ |
|---|---|---|---|
| 7.45 | 25 | 65 | 17 |

## ACID-BASE ANALYSIS*

Step 1: This pH is alkalotic.

Step 2: The calculated pH = 7.55.

Step 3: Both calculated and measured pH are alkalotic; therefore this ABG analysis shows respiratory alkalosis.

Step 4: Compensation for an acute 15 mm Hg decrease in $P_{CO_2}$ would result in about a 3.5 to 4.0 mEq/L decrease in $HCO_3^-$. A chronic 15 mm Hg decrease in $P_{CO_2}$ should result in a decrease of about 7.5 mEq/L or $HCO_3^-$ ~16.5. This ABG analysis reveals chronic respiratory alkalosis.

This patient's acid-base disorder now becomes clearer. Because of his acute asthma, he hyperventilated. Over the more than 24 hours prior to reaching the emergency department, he continued to hyperventilate, and renal compensation occurred. While in the emergency department, the patient developed respiratory failure. Because his bicarbonate buffer reserves were depleted in response to the primary respiratory alkalosis, the secondary acute respiratory failure caused severe acidosis. The earlier ABG analysis did not represent combined respiratory and metabolic acidosis. With this clinical information, you can correctly diagnose acute respiratory acidosis superimposed on chronic respiratory alkalosis. In this clinical setting, an elevated $P_{CO_2}$ is ominous.

The patient was expeditiously intubated and placed on mechanical ventilation. He eventually required general (inhalational) anesthesia with halothane to reverse the bronchospasm. His original ABG analysis showed a mixed disorder of acute respiratory acidosis and chronic respiratory alkalosis.

---

*Analysis of the 12:32 PM ABG data.

CHAPTER 24

# Acute Renal Failure

Mark E. Rosenberg

## CASE 1

A 33-year-old construction worker was admitted to the SICU following a crush injury to his lower extremities. The patient's legs had been caught under debris following a collapse at a construction site. Rescue crews freed him after 4 hours. On examination in the emergency room, his blood pressure was 90/60 and pulse was 110. Extensive soft tissue injury was present in his lower extremities, and x-ray films revealed fractures of both femurs. Initial laboratory findings were as follows: WBC, 11,300/mm$^3$; Hb, 9.7 g/dl; sodium, 137 mEq/L; potassium, 6.2 mEq/L; chloride, 105 mEq/L; $HCO_3^-$, 21 mEq/L; BUN, 23 mg/dl; creatinine, 1.7 mg/dl; calcium, 8.7 mg/dl; phosphorus, 6.5 mg/dl; uric acid, 10 mg/dl. Urine analysis on the small amount of urine obtained after bladder catheterization revealed brown color, a pH of 4.8, 4+ blood, negative protein, and 0 to 2 RBC and pigmented granular casts on microscopic examination. The serum CPK was 20,390 IU/L, and aldolase was 130 U/L. An ECG revealed peaked T waves and occasional multifocal premature ventricular contractions.

The combination of traumatic muscle injury, early elevation in the serum creatinine concentration, increased muscle enzymes, and a positive result on the urine dipstick test for blood in the absence of RBCs on microscopic examination of the urine points to a diagnosis of myoglobinuric acute renal failure secondary to rhabdomyolysis. The reagent for blood on the urinary dipstick will give a positive reaction not only in the presence of RBCs but also with heme pigments such as myoglobin and hemoglobin. Specific tests for urinary or serum myoglobin are available. Following destruction of skeletal muscle either by trauma, as in the current case, or by nontraumatic causes, such as hypophosphatemia, hypokalemia, or polymyositis, large amounts of myoglobin are released into the circulation. Myoglobin consists of a heme pigment contained in a globin chain. The toxicity of myoglobin is thought to reside in the iron-containing heme, which easily dissociates from the globin chain in the acid milieu of the proximal tubule. Other factors that play a causative role in myoglobinuric renal failure are volume depletion (present in this patient because of fluid shifts into damaged muscle and blood loss), fibrin deposition in glomeruli, and increased uric acid production from purines released from injured muscle. Renal vasoconstriction as a result of inhibiting endothelial relaxing factor also may play a role in causing renal failure.

---

This chapter can be studied in conjunction with *Essentials of Surgical Critical Care,* edited by Jerome H. Abrams and Frank B. Cerra (St. Louis: Quality Medical Publishing, Inc., 1993), Chapters 5, 9, *30,* and 31. Italicized number indicates the main chapter reference.

The emergency treatment of rhabdomyolysis is volume repletion and urinary alkalinization. Intravenous infusion of large amounts of normal saline solution or other volume expanders will reverse the prerenal defect caused by fluid shifts and blood loss. The rationale for alkali therapy is to prevent the dissociation of heme from globin and therefore to prevent the direct nephrotoxicity of heme. Mannitol and/or loop diuretics such as furosemide also have been used, although direct proof of their efficacy is lacking. Theoretically, these agents may help relieve intratubular obstruction. Therapy should be started as soon as possible, even at the site of the accident once the patient's trapped limbs are extricated. Therapy of rhabdomyolysis includes:

1. Restoration of circulating volume: normal saline solution (or other volume expander) at 200 to 300 ml/hr following clinical signs and central pressures.
2. Urinary alkalinization: two ampules of sodium bicarbonate (50 ml/ampule) added to 1 L of $D_5W$ and infused at 250 ml/hr for 4 hours.
3. Mannitol: 25 g mannitol can be added to the $D_5W$-bicarbonate solution.

In addition to the release of myoglobin, other intracellular solutes released are potassium, phosphorus, and purines, which are converted to uric acid. The most life-threatening complication of rhabdomyolysis is hyperkalemia because of the potential for inducing cardiac dysrhythmias. The peaked T waves and multifocal premature ventricular contractions (PVCs) are consistent with hyperkalemia. Emergency treatment of hyperkalemia should be instituted in this patient. Intravenous infusion of 10 ml of 10% calcium gluconate will directly antagonize the cardiac and neuromuscular effects of potassium. The onset of action of calcium is immediate but of short duration. Infusion of glucose and insulin will drive potassium into cells. Fifty ml of 50% glucose with 10 units of regular insulin can be infused. This therapy has an onset of action of several minutes and an effect that lasts for approximately 1 hour. More long-term treatment of hyperkalemia can be instituted by administering a potassium-binding resin (e.g., sodium polystyrene sulfonate (Kayexalate) 30 g with 100 ml of 20% sorbitol by mouth). This therapy will remove potassium by exchange for sodium.

A central venous pressure (CVP) catheter was inserted, which revealed a pressure of 4 cm $H_2O$. The patient was treated with 2 L of normal saline solution and two units of packed RBCs. He was taken to the operating room where internal fixation of his fractures and debridement of his leg wounds were performed. Postoperatively the patient's urine output was 15 ml/hr. On examination, BP was 130/85, pulse 100 with multifocal PVCs, CVP 14 cm $H_2O$. Jugular venous pulse was elevated, rales were heard at both lung bases, and an $S_3$ gallop was present. Good distal pulses were present in the lower extremities. The following laboratory values were obtained the next morning: WBC count of 8000/mm$^3$; Hb, 12.2 g/dl; sodium, 131 mEq/L; potassium, 6.5 mEq/L; chloride, 100 mEq/L; $HCO_3^-$ 18; BUN, 37 mg/dl; creatinine, 3.2 mg/dl; calcium, 8 mg/dl; phosphorus, 10.5 mg/dl; uric acid, 14 mg/dl; urine sodium, 70 mEq/L; fractional excretion of sodium (FENa) 2.3%. Results of urine and serum tests were positive for myoglobin.

This patient had developed acute renal failure. The differential diagnosis includes prerenal, postrenal, and intrinsic renal causes. If urinary obstruction is suspected, a urinary catheter should be placed and a renal ultrasound should be performed. In this case both gave negative results. The main differential is between prerenal acute renal failure and acute tubular necrosis (ATN). No clinical evidence for volume depletion was present. In fact, the physical examination and elevated CVP are consistent with fluid overload. This patient most likely had ATN. This is confirmed by the elevated urinary sodium and FENa. Urinary sodium should be low (<20 mEq/L) in the presence of volume depletion and intact tubular function. Therefore the diagnosis of myoglobinuric acute renal failure secondary to rhabdomyolysis could be made. Another clue to this diagnosis is the rapid rise in serum creatinine. In ATN of other causes, the serum creatinine increases approximately 1 mg/dl/day. A much greater rate of increase in serum creatinine occurs following rhabdomyolysis because of muscle breakdown and release of creatine, which undergoes nonenzymatic hydrolysis to creatinine. Further, with rhabdomyolysis, hyperkalemia, hyperphosphatemia, hypocalcemia, and metabolic acidosis may be present before a rise in BUN or creatinine occurs.

Several indications to start dialysis are present. These include fluid overload, hyperkalemia, and acidosis. The elevation in serum phosphorus and uric acid are "softer" indications. Because of the marked tissue catabolism present in rhabdomyolysis, more frequent dialysis often is needed in the initial stages. Hemodialysis should be started in this patient following placement of a double-lumen subclavian catheter for vascular access. An alternative to hemodialysis is continuous arteriovenous hemofiltration with dialysis, which can provide greater solute removal. The oliguric phase of myoglobinuric acute renal failure usually lasts for 7 to 10 days, after which the urine output should start to increase and the BUN and creatinine should decrease.

The patient must be observed closely for the development of a compartment syndrome since injured muscle swells in a potentially confined space. Such swelling can result in permanent ischemic or nerve damage to the affected limb, and also cause a second wave of rhabdomyolysis with consequent loss of any remaining renal function.

> After 2 weeks of dialysis support, the urine output increased, followed several days later by a decrease in BUN and creatinine concentrations. During the recovery phase, the following laboratory values were obtained: calcium, 12.3 mg/dl; phosphorus, 5.2 mg/dl; and creatinine, 2 mg/dl.

One of the complications observed during the recovery phase of myoglobinuric renal failure is the development of hypercalcemia. During the injury phase, calcium is deposited in the necrotic muscle. This process is accelerated by the elevated calcium-phosphorus product found in the early stages of rhabdomyolysis. As the injured muscle heals, the calcium is resorbed, in some cases leading to hypercalcemia. Other factors that may contribute to the elevated calcium are increased parathyroid hormone and vitamin D. If symptoms of hypercalcemia develop, therapy will be needed. In the patient with established diuresis, this therapy can consist of normal saline solution and furosemide. If a patient is still undergoing dialysis, lowering the dialysate calcium concentration will facilitate diffusive calcium loss.

## CASE 2

> A 74-year-old woman was admitted to the hospital with dizziness and midabdominal pain. Her history was remarkable for hypertension of 20 years' duration, a myocardial infarct 4 years earlier, and diabetes treated for the preceding 4 years with an oral hypoglycemic agent. On examination her blood pressure was 90/60; pulse, 120; temperature, 98.6° F. Her jugular venous pulse was not well noted. Lungs were clear and heart sounds normal. Abdominal examination revealed an 8 cm pulsating mass located in the midabdomen. Distal pulses were decreased bilaterally. The following laboratory values were obtained: WBC count, 8200/mm$^3$; Hb, 8.6 g/dl; platelets, 250,000/mm$^3$; sodium, 140 mEq/L; potassium, 4.6 mEq/L; chloride, 104 mEq/L; $HCO_3^-$, 24 mEq/L; BUN, 23 mg/dl; creatinine, 1.4 mg/dl; and results of the urine analysis were normal. An abdominal ultrasound confirmed the clinical diagnosis of a ruptured aortic aneurysm.

Emergency surgical therapy is required in this patient. She has several risk factors for the development of acute renal failure in the perioperative period, including old age, underlying cardiac disease, diabetes, volume depletion, and the need for major cardiovascular surgery. She also has underlying renal insufficiency. The creatinine clearance can be estimated by the Cockroft and Gault formula:

$$\text{CrCl (ml/min)} = [(140 - \text{Age}) \times \text{Lean body weight}]/[\text{PCr} \times 72] \times 0.85$$

Based on the patient's weight of 58 kg, her estimated creatinine clearance is 32 ml/min. The decreased creatinine clearance emphasizes the need to factor body weight and age into the interpretation of serum creatinine concentration. In preparation for surgery, a pulmonary artery catheter should be inserted for measurement of filling pressures to aid in perioperative fluid management. Aggressive fluid therapy should be instituted with normal saline solution and packed RBCs (when they become available). Evidence suggests that mannitol or loop diuretics may provide prophylaxis against acute renal failure during aortic aneurysm surgery. Since severe volume depletion is present in this patient, these agents should be avoided until her volume status is restored.

> The initial pulmonary capillary wedge pressure (PCWP) was 4 mm Hg. As the operating room was being prepared, 2 L of normal saline solution was infused along with two units of packed RBCs. Fluid therapy raised the PCWP to 10 mm Hg. A ruptured aortic aneurysm was found at surgery with its origin just below the takeoff of the renal arteries. A vascular clamp was placed below the renal arteries, and an aortoiliac bypass was performed. Two episodes of severe hypotension that occurred during surgery responded to fluid resuscitation. The urine output during the 4-hour surgery averaged 20 ml/hr. The patient was transferred to the SICU. Five hours after the surgery, the SICU resident was called because of the patient's persistent oliguria, which averaged 20 ml/min. On examination, blood pressure was 90/70 mm Hg; pulse, 120 and regular; and PCWP, 4 mm Hg. The lungs were clear and heart sounds normal. The patient's abdomen was diffusely tender, but the wound was intact. Distal pulses were present bilaterally. The following laboratory values were obtained: WBC count, 9800/mm$^3$; Hb, 9.7 g/dl; sodium, 144 mEq/L; potassium, 4.8 mEq/L; chloride, 106 mEq/L; $HCO_3^-$, 21 mEq/L; BUN, 38 mg/dl; creatinine, 1.8 mg/dl. Urine analysis showed specific gravity of 1.028, trace protein, but negative microscopic examination. Urine sodium was 6 mEq/L, and the FENa was 0.3%.

The approach to the oliguria and elevated BUN and creatinine concentrations should include an assessment of prerenal, postrenal, and renal factors. Because of the potential risk of ureteric ligation during surgery, a renal ultrasound examination should be obtained. It is possible that obstruction can be present, but dilatation may not have occurred. If results of the initial ultrasound examination are negative and the index of suspicion is high, the ultrasound can be repeated in 24 to 48 hours. The main differential diagnosis in this patient is between prerenal acute renal failure and ATN. ATN secondary to renal ischemia is possible in this patient, especially in view of the preoperative and intraoperative hypotension. However, the examination and urinary indexes favor the diagnosis of prerenal acute renal failure. The PCWP is low, there is an elevation in the BUN-to-creatinine ratio, and the urine examination suggests good tubular function (as evidenced by the avid water and sodium reabsorption that occurs as a consequence of the prerenal state). This reabsorption is manifest as a high urine specific gravity and low urine sodium and FENa.

Fluid therapy is necessary to reverse the prerenal state. This therapy consists of normal saline solution, other volume expanders, and/or packed RBCs. Despite the oliguria, diuretics are not indicated because of the underlying volume depletion. The physical examinations, PCWP, urine output, and electrolyte concentrations should be followed as markers of response to fluid therapy.

With appropriate fluid therapy, the PCWP increased to 12 mm Hg and the urine output rose to 70 ml/min. The following morning the serum creatinine concentration was 1.4 mg/dl. The next day, the patient developed fever to 103° F and hypotension with a blood pressure of 70/60. The PCWP was 4 mm Hg, cardiac output was elevated, and systemic vascular resistance was decreased. Cultures were obtained, and the patient was started on broad-spectrum antibiotics. Despite aggressive fluid therapy, the patient remained hypotensive, which necessitated the use of dopamine, which was titrated up to a dose of 12 μg/kg/min in order to maintain a systolic blood pressure above 100. Over the ensuing 24 hours, a total of 10 L of intravenous fluid was administered to maintain the PCWP between 6 and 10 mm Hg. During this time the urine output was 15 to 20 ml/hr. Laboratory evaluation results were as follows: WBC count, 23,400/$mm^3$ with a left shift; Hb, 11.8 g/dl; platelets, 123,000/$mm^3$; sodium, 136 mEq/L; potassium, 5 mEq/L; chloride, 110 mEq/L; $HCO_3^-$, 13 mEq/L; BUN, 46 mg/dl; creatinine, 2.4 mg/dl; glucose, 160 mg/dl; urine sodium, 60 mEq/L; FENa, 2.5%. Urine analysis showed specific gravity of 1.005, trace protein, 1+ blood, 4 to 6 RBCs, 5 to 7 renal tubular epithelial cells, 4 to 6 granular casts. Blood cultures were positive for a Gram-negative rod.

The patient had developed Gram-negative sepsis. Renal ischemia secondary to renal hypoperfusion had led to acute renal failure. The decreased renal perfusion was caused by sepsis and vasoconstrictor doses of dopamine, which were needed to maintain blood pressure. The low urine specific gravity and elevated urine sodium and FENa suggested that tubular function was no longer intact. Also, on microscopic examination of the urine, RBCs, renal tubular epithelial cells, and granular casts were present. Therefore the clinical picture was consistent with a diagnosis of ATN. ATN developed despite appropriate therapy with fluid and antibiotics. At this stage, the return of renal function must await regeneration of renal tubular epithelial cells, a process that may take several weeks. The most important prognostic factor for return of renal function is to gain control of the underlying septic process. At present, no indications for dialysis are present. However, careful attention needs to be paid to the patient's fluid and electrolyte state and dialysis initiated when indications develop.

SECTION 5 *Gastrointestinal and Hepatic Function*

# CHAPTER 25

# *Physiologic Alterations of the Gut Mucosal Barrier*

David C. Evans • Oren K. Steinmetz • Jonathan L. Meakins

## CASE 1

A 47-year-old man was admitted to the SICU for what appears to be subacute rejection 18 days following left renal transplantation for end-stage diabetic nephropathy. Immunotherapy, including azathioprine, cyclosporine, and prednisone, was maximized and hemodynamic monitoring was initiated. The patient appeared to be in mild distress, with renal function having deteriorated slowly over the preceding few days. The following clinical measurements were obtained: pulse 115 beats/min; respiratory rate, 26 breaths/min; blood pressure, 105/60 mm Hg; temperature, 38.2° C (100.8° F); cardiac index, 5.5 L/min/$m^2$; systemic vascular resistance, 870 dyne · sec · $cm^{-5}$; urine output, 60 ml/hr; and serum creatinine, 350 mmol/L. Due to long-standing ileus, total parenteral nutrition was administered through a central venous catheter. A urinary catheter and nasogastric tube were both placed.

Two days later the patient's condition had worsened: pulse, 130 beats/min; respiratory rate, 32 breaths/min; blood pressure, 90/45 mm Hg; temperature, 39.1° C (102.38° F); cardiac index, 7.4 L/min/$m^2$; systemic vascular resistance, 440 dyne · sec · $cm^{-5}$; urine output, negligible; and serum creatinine, 650 mmol/L. Clinically, the patient was lethargic with a moderately distended and quiet abdomen. An ileus pattern persists on x-ray film.

- *Outline an approach to the management of the patient at this point. What is the underlying pathologic condition likely to be?*

The patient is clearly manifesting a hyperdynamic or "septic" response to some inciting stimulus. As with any febrile postoperative patient presenting with this clinical picture, systemic infection must be considered, and its source must be urgently sought. Blood, sputum, urine, and wound cultures should be obtained, and broad-spectrum antibiotics should be begun. The central line should be removed, and its tip should be cultured.

Acute rejection of the transplanted kidney is the other likely explanation for the patient's

This chapter can be studied in conjunction with *Essentials of Surgical Critical Care,* edited by Jerome H. Abrams and Frank B. Cerra (St. Louis: Quality Medical Publishing, Inc., 1993), Chapters 2, *32,* 34, and 47. Italicized number indicates the main chapter reference.

clinical deterioration. If adequate fluid resuscitation fails to prompt a satisfactory urine output, the serum creatinine concentration continues to increase, and percutaneous biopsies are histologically compatible with fulminant rejection, the transplanted kidney should be removed and dialysis should be initiated.

Since these conditions were present with this patient, a nephrectomy was appropriately performed. Two days postoperatively the patient was still markedly febrile but somewhat improved clinically: temperature, 38.7° C (101.66° F); pulse, 110 beats/min; respirations, 22 breaths/min; blood pressure, 110/65 mm Hg; cardiac index, 5.1 L/min/$m^2$; systemic vascular resistance, 1200 dyne · sec · $cm^{-5}$. Dialysis was performed to ensure appropriate fluid and electrolyte balance. Blood cultures drawn previously were noted as positive for *Candida albicans*.

- *What might explain this result?*

Rejection as a primary process induces a systemic "septic" response mediated by a host of cytokines and other cellular macromolecules, which are the common final pathway in many infectious and noninfectious conditions that may lead to multiple system organ failure. Removal of the ailing organ addresses the primary process and thereby ameliorates the body's septic response. However, just as disseminated intravascular coagulation, adult respiratory distress syndrome, and acute tubular necrosis represent well recognized syndromes of system failure under these conditions, the gut must be considered susceptible to decompensation. Sloughing of mucosa with superficial necrosis, edema, and failure of tight junctions are documented changes.

Since transplant patients, particularly those experiencing organ rejection, are severely immunosuppressed, host defenses often are unable to contain both exogenous and endogenous sources of microbial infection. Debilitation of gut associated lymphocytic tissue (GALT) permits mucosal translocation of enteric organisms and toxins, which then can initiate a cascade of events culminating in multiple system organ failure. In this individual, in whom the prolonged use of intravenous hyperalimentation has rendered intestinal villus height decreased, enterocyte mass reduced, and brush border enzymes less active, gut barrier function is further impaired. Ileus and distention are unreliable clinical signs of gut dysfunction. *Candida albicans* is a skin and gut saprophyte that commonly produces fungemia in immunocompromised hosts. Impaired immunity, enterocyte compromise, and possibly an altered balance of microflora from antibiotic use may facilitate hematogenous monilial invasion from the gut.

Appropriate therapeutic measures would include systemic antifungal therapy (amphotericin B and flucytosine), cessation of administration of antibacterial agents, reduction of use of immunosuppressive agents, and early transition from parenteral to enteral (glutamine-enriched) alimentation as a means of restoring the physical component of the gut mucosal barrier.

## CASE 2

A 65-year-old woman known for heavy smoking and alcohol abuse presented to the emergency department with abdominal pain, tachycardia, and hypotension. Examination revealed confusion, diaphoresis, and discolored flanks. The following clinical measurements were obtained: pulse, 140 beats/min; respiratory rate, 34 breaths/min; blood pressure, 85/40 mm Hg; temperature, 36.5° C (97.7° F); $Po_2$, 55 mm Hg; $Pco_2$, 45 mm Hg; and pH, 7.22. An elevated serum amylase concentration prompted doing a CT scan, which demonstrated severe pancreatic inflammation. Hemorrhagic pancreatitis was diagnosed, and the patient was admitted to the SICU for management.

Twelve hours later, 8 L of crystalloid and three units of packed RBCs had only marginally improved the patient's hemodynamic status. Nonoliguric acute tubular necrosis had developed, and the patient required intubation and ventilation.

- *What is appropriate management in this situation? How can one best minimize the risk of gut mucosal barrier breakdown and ensuing multiple system organ failure?*

Pancreatitis is a well-acknowledged initiator of a hyperdynamic (septic) response, which may lead to multiple system organ failure. Prognosis has been related to Ranson's criteria (see box, p. 126), which should be ascertained for the first 48-hour period. Immediate, vigorous, and effective resuscitation must be performed in order to ensure the best possible outcome. Volume replacement with blood and crystalloid, maximized oxygen delivery employing mechanical ventilation and supplemental oxygen as needed, and hemodynamic monitoring all should be instituted. Preservation of the gut mucosal barrier requires adequate splanchnic perfusion, which is best achieved by prompt resuscitation. It is likely that this patient already has endured some degree of intestinal hypoperfusion. The relative intestinal ischemia probably is exacerbated by an underlying vascular insufficiency, a consequence of her extensive smoking history. This patient is at particular risk for gut bacterial translocation. Low-dose dopamine or calcium channel-blocking agents (if hemodynamic stability has been achieved) are pharmacologic aids that may improve splanchnic blood flow and therefore should be considered.

Poor nutrition and impaired immunity are anticipated in the alcoholic and should be rectified as far as possible with parenteral hyperalimentation. Supplementation with 2% glutamine is gaining acceptance as a mode of supporting the nutritive needs of the intestinal enterocyte. Some concern remains about the stability of glutamine in solution and the potential toxicity of its metabolites. These issues have not been fully resolved and require further study.

Good evidence exists to forego nasogastric suction in pancreatitis if vomiting and distension are absent. Nasogastric decompression does not minimize pancreatic stimulation in a manner that alters outcome; yet it does compromise the lower esophageal sphincter and predisposes to aspiration. Particularly when nasogastric tube placement is required, sucralfate, rather than antacid therapy, is the best protection against erosive gastritis and stress ulceration. Sucralfate maintains normal gastric acidity, which, in turn, reduces bacterial colonization of the stomach. The risk of aspiration pneumonia appears to be reduced.

Treating the primary process in order to abate the "septic" response requires appropriate management of the inflamed and necrotic pancreas. Although the use of subcutaneous somatostatin may improve outcome by reducing pancreatic exocrine function, aggressive surgical debridement of the pancreatic bed is more urgently required in this patient to limit ongoing tissue destruction and to stem the release of acute-phase reactants and other mediators of the septic response. These mediators collectively compromise gut mocosal epithelium and theoretically result in dysfunction of other organ systems. There is no identified role for antibiotic prophylaxis in acute pancreatitis. Repeated cultures of all body fluids should be diligently obtained since infection of enteric or other origin is a definite risk in all critically ill patients.

# CHAPTER 26

# *Acute Gastrointestinal Hemorrhage*

Jerome H. Abrams

## CASE

A 73-year-old man was admitted for left lower quadrant abdominal pain and fever. Pain was described as crampy with localization to the left lower quadrant over the 24 hours prior to admission. The patient reported feeling feverish. He had had a markedly reduced appetite, denied vomiting, and had not been able to pass stool or flatus for 24 hours. His medical history was remarkable for significant alcohol consumption. He stated, and his family verified, that he had not consumed alcoholic beverages for the 12 years prior to this admission.

Physical examination revealed a moderately obese gentleman. His temperature was 102.3° F. Blood pressure was 140/75, heart rate was 110, and respiratory rate was 14. The physical examination was unremarkable except for abdominal findings. Left lower quadrant tenderness with involuntary guarding was noted. Bowel sounds were not detected. The patient had no evidence for ascites, the liver was not palpable, and no other stigmata of chronic liver failure were noted. With a diagnosis of acute diverticulitis, he was admitted for nasogastric suction and treatment with broad-spectrum antibiotics. Over the next 24 hours, the patient's tenderness increased and his fever persisted.

Having failed conservative management, the patient was taken to the operating room with a preoperative diagnosis of acute diverticulitis. On abdominal exploration, the sigmoid colon was found to be acutely inflamed. The remainder of the abdominal exploration demonstrated a firm liver, consistent with cirrhosis. A sigmoid resection was performed. An end-on colostomy and Hartmann's pouch were fashioned. The patient recovered well from this procedure and was discharged to home on postoperative day 8.

Three months following this procedure, the patient was admitted for an elective take-down of his colostomy. The colostomy take-down proceeded uneventfully. The patient did well until postoperative day 2, at which time a small amount of hematemesis was noted. The patient required two units of packed RBC transfusion. Following transfusion, his hemoglobin remained stable, and he had no additional evidence of acute gastrointestinal hemorrhage. Forty-eight hours following his first bleeding episode, on postoperative day 4, he passed melanotic stool and required three units of packed RBC transfusion. With these findings, the patient was transferred to your hospital.

- *What is your approach to the patient at this time?*

---

This chapter can be studied in conjunction with *Essentials of Surgical Critical Care,* edited by Jerome H. Abrams and Frank B. Cerra (St. Louis: Quality Medical Publishing, Inc., 1993), Chapters 2 and *33*. Italicized number indicates the main chapter reference.

The patient has acute gastrointestinal hemorrhage. His hematemesis, occurring a few days prior to his transfer, is consistent with an upper GI source. The patient has also passed melanotic stool without any additional evidence of hematemesis. His history of chronic alcohol abuse and the operative findings consistent with cirrhosis of the liver raise the concern of esophageal varices as the source of bleeding. Since the patient required five units of packed RBCs prior to transfer, an accurate diagnosis is necessary for optimum therapy. In particular, if the patient's current bleeding source is from the lower GI tract, a transfusion requirement of four units or greater in a 24-hour period places this patient at a higher probability for requiring emergency surgery. A determination of whether the bleeding source is from the upper or lower GI tract is the first step. Accordingly, upper GI endoscopy is performed.

> Upper GI endoscopy findings revealed the presence of esophageal varices. At the time of the examination, no bleeding from the varices was observed. Pooling of blood in the stomach was observed and was removed by suction. Evidence of mild gastritis was noted. The duodenum was examined, and a blood clot was adherent to the duodenal wall. This clot, however, was easily removed with a pressurized stream of fluid, and no evidence of ulcer disease was identified. After endoscopic examination, the impression was the presence of mild gastritis, esophageal varices, and no evidence of bleeding from the varices. The presumed cause of bleeding was gastritis. With the findings of pooling of blood in the stomach and evidence of gastritis, $H_2$-blockers and antacids were administered. The patient remained stable for 12 hours and then passed stool containing dark blood. His hemoglobin decreased by 2 g/dl, and he required transfusion of two additional units of packed RBCs.
>
> - *What is your evaluation at this time?*

Evidence of acute blood loss is again present. The patient has now required a total of seven units of packed RBC transfusion. With the evidence of varices on the initial upper GI examination, the question of bleeding from the varices remains. If the patient should have acute variceal bleeding, consideration should be given to sclerotherapy. With acute bleeding, many clinicians would favor sclerotherapy, which has a reasonable expectation of controlling bleeding. If sclerotherapy is not possible or is unsuccessful, the use of a Sengstaken-Blakemore tube can be of benefit in temporarily controlling the bleeding. Clearly, an accurate diagnosis is necessary for appropriate therapy. Accordingly, a repeat upper GI endoscopy is performed to evaluate the possibility of bleeding from either gastritis or varices.

> On the second upper GI endoscopic examination, the varices were again noted. Again, the endoscopist observed no bleeding from the varices. Examination of the varices included a careful retroflexed view to facilitate evaluation of the varices from all aspects. The gastritis had resolved. No evidence of blood in the stomach was found. Repeat examination of the duodenum revealed no abnormality.

Despite evidence of blood loss, no convincing site of bleeding from the upper GI tract has been identified. This patient has had a large transfusion requirement, and establishing a diagnosis remains of great importance. In the absence of an upper GI source, is a lower GI source possible? In particular, could the patient's new surgical anastomosis be the source of continuing hemorrhage? Evaluation of the patient for a lower GI bleeding source is the next priority. Colonoscopy might be a satisfactory diagnostic approach, but colonoscopy in the presence of acute bleeding can be difficult. In addition, colonoscopy poses a risk to the newly formed surgical anastomosis. Two other possible diagnostic procedures are angiography and the use of the radionuclide tagged–red cell scan. The selection of tests depends on the estimated rate of bleeding. This patient has required approximately two units of blood over 24 hours. The rate of bleeding is probably not sufficient to make angiography likely to reveal the diagnosis. Accordingly, a tagged–red cell study is obtained. This type of study can detect a lower rate of bleeding than can angiography because it does not depend on the presence of active bleeding at the moment that the angiographic contrast is injected. The RBCs circulate, and repeat studies can be obtained over 24 to 36 hours.

> The tagged–red cell study was obtained and revealed that radioactive counts appeared in an area consistent with the left colon soon after the tagged red cells were injected. Radioactive counts accumulated in a structure that was consistent with the descending sigmoid colon. The patient's passage of melanotic stool in the nuclear medicine department caused the counts to disappear.

The tagged–red cell study suggests a left colon source. The patient now has evidence for a colonic source. Is the colonic source likely to explain all of the findings? In particular, can pooling of blood in the stomach be explained by a left colon source? In this situation, not all of the bleeding can be attributed to the colon. Since the patient has significant risk associated with surgical exploration because of the cirrhosis and the high probability of dense adhesions, you decide to attempt colonoscopy and coagulation of the bleeding site, if possible. While preparing for the colonoscopic procedure, you begin an infusion of vasopressin.

> With evidence for a colonic bleeding source, intravenous vasopressin was begun. Before colonoscopy was performed, the patient vomited a small amount of blood and passed a large amount of melanotic stool. He required five units of packed RBC transfusion and was hypotensive.
>
> - *What is your approach at this time?*

The patient is currently on vasopressin and has new evidence of bleeding. Findings now include hematemesis and a large amount of melanotic stool. With a colonic source of bleeding already identified, the colon remains a likely source of hemorrhage at this time. Nonetheless, how can one account for hematemesis from a distal colon bleeding source? Accordingly, emergency upper GI endoscopy is performed to again evaluate the varices.

> At this examination, evidence for variceal bleeding was encountered.
>
> - *What is your approach at this point?*

The bleeding varices may very well account for the most recent episode of bleeding. The discovery of bleeding varices, however, does not rule out additional bleeding from the colon. To control the bleeding varices, a Sengstaken-Blakemore tube is placed carefully, and the gastric and the esophageal balloons are inflated according to protocol. Because the possibility of continued colonic bleeding exists and the patient has sufficient transfusion requirement to make angiography likely to disclose the source of bleeding if it were from the colon, an angiogram is considered. With return of blood pressure and pulse to stable values through the use of a Sengstaken-Blakemore tube, the patient is transferred to the angiography suite. Angiography fails to reveal a bleeding site, and the conclusion is that the patient's most acute episode is from the bleeding varices.

> The patient's condition was stabilized over the next 24 hours. The Sengstaken-Blakemore tube was removed and the patient's bleeding ceased. The patient underwent variceal sclerotherapy successfully. He had no further episodes of colonic bleeding and was discharged to home.

# CHAPTER 27

## *Pancreatitis*

**Barry W. Feig**

### CASE 1

A 42-year-old man with a history of heavy alcohol consumption over several years presented to the emergency room with complaints of epigastric pain radiating to the middle of his back. He had had several episodes of bile-stained emesis. The patient denied any fever or chills. The patient's pain had been constant and severe, waking him up from sleep early that morning. He had been admitted to other hospitals on two prior occasions for similar episodes of pain. On physical examination, the patient's temperature was 99.8° F, his pulse was 96 beats/min, and his respiratory rate was 22 breaths/min. Breath sounds were clear and noted bilaterally. The patient's abdomen was soft and slightly distended, and bowel sounds were absent. Tenderness to palpation in the upper abdomen with voluntary guarding was noted.

- *How would you proceed with the initial evaluation of this patient?*

This patient has signs and symptoms consistent with an acute abdominal process. At this point the differential diagnosis would include acute cholecystitis, peptic ulcer disease, perforated viscus, acute appendicitis, and acute pancreatitis. The initial evaluation should include an upright CXR film, supine and upright abdominal x-ray films, CBC, electrolytes, calcium, blood urea nitrogen, creatinine, amylase, LDH, and SGOT.

An abdominal flat plate and upright x-ray examination was obtained. It showed a dilated loop of small intestine in the left upper quadrant of the abdomen. No free air was present under the diaphragm on upright CXR film. Laboratory studies showed the following values:

| WBC | Hb | K | Mg | Ca | Glu | $Po_2$ | BUN | $CO_2$ | LDH | SGOT | Amyl |
|---|---|---|---|---|---|---|---|---|---|---|---|
| 12,200 | 13.5 | 3 | 1.6 | 8.2 | 157 | 82 | 16 | 26 | 152 | 75 | 875 |

Based on these findings, a presumptive diagnosis of acute pancreatitis is made. The patient's

This chapter can be studied in conjunction with *Essentials of Surgical Critical Care,* edited by Jerome H. Abrams and Frank B. Cerra (St. Louis: Quality Medical Publishing, Inc., 1993), Chapters 1, 2, 20, 27, and *34.* Italicized number indicates the main chapter reference.

condition does not appear to be a severe, complicated case of pancreatitis from the clinical and laboratory data accrued thus far.

- *How would you proceed with patient management?*

The patient was admitted to the ward. An IV infusion of 5% dextrose in lactated Ringer's solution was started, and the patient was allowed nothing by mouth. Vital signs and urine output were strictly monitored every 4 hours. Potassium and magnesium supplementation was given intravenously to replace serum deficits. Urine output was 500 ml for the first 8 hours, and adequate pain control was achieved with IV ketorolac tromethamine. Repeat laboratory studies 12 hours after admission were as follows:

| WBC | Hb | K | Ca | Glu | $Po_2$ | BUN | LDH | SGOT | Amyl | Lac |
|---|---|---|---|---|---|---|---|---|---|---|
| 9600 | 12.7 | 3.6 | 8 | 138 | 98 | 10 | 102 | 35 | 652 | 1.1 |

On physical examination, the abdomen was soft, with hypoactive bowel sounds and mild tenderness to palpation noted in the epigastric region. Subjectively, this patient had decreased abdominal pain without any nausea or emesis.

The laboratory and clinical data obtained indicate that the patient is improving with supportive therapy. Therefore supportive treatment should be continued along with careful monitoring of the patient.

Six hours later, the patient complained of severe abdominal pain in the epigastric region radiating to the back. The pain was not relieved by IV administration of meperidine. Repeat laboratory examination gave the following values:

| WBC | Hb | Ca | $Po_2$ | BUN | LDH | SGOT | Amyl | Lac |
|---|---|---|---|---|---|---|---|---|
| 9800 | 12.2 | 8.1 | 87 | 12 | 139 | 60 | 975 | 1.6 |

A CT scan was obtained and showed a homogeneous, edematous pancreas. The gland demonstrated uniform enhancement with intravenous contrast. No peripancreatic loculated fluid collections were present.

The CT scan confirms the diagnosis of acute uncomplicated pancreatitis. Only minimal change has occurred in the patient's laboratory studies. Supportive treatment should be continued at this point.

The patient's pain gradually improved over the next 12 hours, and again minimal abdominal tenderness was noted and normal active bowel sounds were present. Repeat laboratory values were:

| WBC | Hb | Ca | BUN | LDH | SGOT | Amyl |
|---|---|---|---|---|---|---|
| 7600 | 12 | 8.5 | 6 | 112 | 37 | 286 |

Both clinical and laboratory evidence of improvement can be noted in this patient's condition. At this point the patient is begun on oral feedings and the IV line is removed. The laboratory examination is repeated on a regular basis until values are normal. When the patient is tolerating a regular diet, he should be discharged and given follow-up treatment for alcohol abuse.

## CASE 2

A 32-year-old woman with no prior medical problems presented with a chief complaint of 2 days of severe upper abdominal pain that was constant and radiated to the back. Recently, she had multiple episodes of nausea and emesis. Her breath sounds were decreased at the bases bilaterally (L>R). The abdomen was distended, and no bowel sounds were noted on auscultation. Tenderness and involuntary guarding were noted in the epigastric region. The patient had a temperature of 100.4° F, a pulse of 125 beats/min, and a respiratory rate of 32 breaths/min. On admission, her blood pressure was 96/62 mm Hg.

This patient presents in a hyperdynamic state as a result of an acute intra-abdominal process. The differential diagnosis and the initial laboratory studies are the same as in the patient in Case 1. A nasogastric tube is placed to treat the ileus and for gastric decompression, with return of 800 ml of coffee-ground material. Placement of a Foley catheter yields 200 ml of urine. An upright CXR shows a moderate left pleural effusion; no free air is noted under the diaphragm. Supine and upright abdominal x-ray films show a paucity of air in the bowel with a generalized ground-glass appearance, consistent with ascitic fluid.

The initial laboratory results were noted as:

| WBC | Hb | K | Mg | Ca | Glu | BUN | LDH | SGOT | Amyl | Trigly | Lac | pH | $Pco_2$ | $Po_2$ |
|---|---|---|---|---|---|---|---|---|---|---|---|---|---|---|
| 16,800 | 14.2 | 3.1 | 1.5 | 4.8 | 257 | 22 | 425 | 297 | 864 | 8224 | 4.6 | 7.46 | 27 | 62 |

One liter of lactated Ringer's solution was administered intravenously. No change occurred in the patients vital signs, and urine output over the next hour was 20 ml.

This patient has at least five of Ranson's criteria (see box), which is consistent with a case of severe pancreatitis. The oliguria is most likely the result of decreased intravascular volume associated with third-space fluid losses. The patient is admitted to the SICU for close observation. A pulmonary artery catheter should be placed, not only to guide the amount of fluid replacement,

### Prognostic Indicators of Severe Pancreatitis*

| *On admission* | *During first 48 hours* |
|---|---|
| Age >55 years | Hematocrit decrease >10% |
| WBC >16,000/mm$^3$ | BUN increase >5 mg/dl |
| Glucose >200 mg/dl | Serum calcium <8 mg/dl |
| LDH >350 IU/L | Arterial $Po_2$ <60 mm Hg |
| SGOT >120 IU/L | Base deficit >4 mEq/L |
| | Fluid sequestration >6 L |

*From Ranson JHC, Rifkind KM, Roses DF, et al. Prognostic signs and the role of operative management in acute pancreatitis. Surg Gynecol Obstet 139:69, 1974. By permission of *Surgery, Gynecology, and Obstetrics.*

but to obtain early restoration of oxygen transport. Electrolyte abnormalities are corrected with infusion of potassium, magnesium, and calcium salts. The patient is begun on an $H_2$-blocker as prophylaxis against stress ulceration, and administration of a second-generation cephalosporin is begun for prophylaxis against secondary bacterial infections.

The data obtained following placement of the pulmonary artery catheter were noted as:

| P | BP | CO/CI | PCWP | $DO_2$ | $VO_2$ | $DVO_2$ | SVR | Lac |
|---|---|---|---|---|---|---|---|---|
| 135 | 90/60 | 5.2/3.1 | 6 | 584 | 132 | 5.2 | 1785 | 4.6 |

Based on these data and the previously noted lactate concentration of 4.6, it is clear that this patient is in a flow-dependent state. The oxygen consumption is well below what is expected for a case of severe pancreatitis, and the increased arteriovenous content difference indicates maximal oxygen extraction.

In view of the low pulmonary capillary wedge pressure (PCWP), the patient was given infusion of additional 2 L of lactated Ringer's solution. In response to this infusion, the PCWP increased to 10 mm Hg, with a cardiac output of 10 L/min and a systemic vascular resistance of 1280 dyne · sec · $cm^{-5}$. The oxygen delivery was then 1345 ml/min with an oxygen consumption of 185 ml/min/$m^2$. The hemoglobin and lactate concentrations both fell, to 11.8 and 2.9, respectively. The pulse remained at 128 beats/min, with a slight increase in the blood pressure to 104/68 mm Hg. The urine output increased to 60 ml over the next 2 hours. After administration of a total of 3 L of crystalloid, some improvement in oxygen transport occurred, but a delivery-independent state was not achieved. An ultrasound examination of the right upper quadrant of the abdomen was performed to assess the gallbladder, biliary tree, and pancreas. No stones were present in the gallbladder, and the common bile duct was 0.8 cm in diameter. No intrahepatic ductal dilation was noted, and the pancreas was obscured by ascitic fluid. At this point the ultrasound examination is important in order to rule out an impacted gallstone in the ampulla of Vater as the cause of the pancreatitis. If such a gallstone were present, an endoscopic sphincterotomy could be performed to relieve the obstruction.

Another 2 L of crystalloid solution was infused, and the following laboratory and hemodynamic measurements were obtained:

| WBC | Hb | K | Ca | Glu | BUN | Lac | pH | $PCO_2$ | $PO_2$ |
|---|---|---|---|---|---|---|---|---|---|
| 17,000 | 9.7 | 3.1 | 5.1 | 225 | 25 | 1.8 | 7.35 | 43 | 57 |

| P | BP | CO/CI | PCWP | $DO_2$ | $VO_2$ | $DVO_2$ | SVR |
|---|---|---|---|---|---|---|---|
| 128 | 102/68 | 12.9/6.7 | 10 | 2015 | 289 | 3.7 | 1150 |

At this point the patient was tachypneic, with a respiratory rate of 36 breaths/min. The abdomen was becoming increasingly distended.

Despite what appears to be a state of flow-independent oxygen consumption, the patient seems to be deteriorating clinically. Because of his worsening respiratory status, the patient is intubated and placed on mechanical ventilatory support. The aggressive fluid resuscitation is maintained to keep the urine output at a minimum of 1 ml/kg/hr. Replacement of electrolytes also is continued. Repeat laboratory examination shows a decrease in amylase concentration to 425

IU/L and a triglyceride concentration of 4375 mg%. The patient is begun on total parenteral hyperalimentation for nutritional support.

> Seventy-two hours after admission to the SICU, the patient had a fever (102.8° F). The abdomen was distended and tense, and the patient remained on mechanical ventilatory support. The following data were obtained:

| P | BP | CO/CI | PCWP | $Do_2$ | $Vo_2$ | SVR | pH | $Pco_2$ | $Po_2$ |
|---|---|---|---|---|---|---|---|---|---|
| 138 | 94/58 | 11.8/6 | 12 | 1990 | 256 | 422 | 7.38 | 36 | 124 |

| WBC | Hb | Ca | Glu | BUN | LDH | SGOT | Amyl | Trigly | Lac |
|---|---|---|---|---|---|---|---|---|---|
| 20,900 | 9.9 | 6.8 | 187 | 22 | 360 | 220 | 289 | 1245 | 1.4 |

> The patient underwent a CT scan of the abdomen. Homogeneous enhancement of the pancreas was seen with an intravenous contrast bolus. A marked amount of ascites was present without any obvious loculated areas. A sample of this fluid was aspirated and sent for Gram's stain and culture. The fluid had the appearance of "crank-case oil" on gross inspection, and the Gram's stain showed no organisms or WBCs.

At this time no indication exists for operative intervention. The patient is continued on supportive treatment, and all other possible sources of fever are evaluated. The hemodynamic data indicate that the patient has been maintained in a state of flow-independent oxygen transport, although at a greatly increased metabolic rate. The patient continues in this persistent hyperdynamic state for another 48 hours. With no improvement in 5 days, the patient is taken to the operating room for exploration.

At exploration, a large amount of dark ascitic fluid is found along with necrotic, devitalized retroperitoneal tissue. This tissue is debrided, and the lesser omental sac is packed open with saline-soaked gauze. During the next 2 weeks, the patient is brought back to the operating room five times for mechanical debridement. During this interval the temperature and signs of hypermetabolism gradually decrease. Oxygen consumption, pulse rate, cardiac output, and ventilatory requirements all decrease. The patient is able to be transferred to the ward 3 weeks following the last exploration.

# CHAPTER 28

# *Acute Abdomen*

**Michael D. Pasquale ▪ Roderick A. Barke**

## CASE 1

A 78-year-old woman presented to the emergency room with complaints of epigastric pain. She stated that she had not been feeling well (anorexia, malaise) for the past several weeks and had developed abdominal pain 3 days prior to admission. She described the pain as initially being a dull ache in the epigastrum. Over the 48 hours prior to her arrival at the emergency department, it had worsened progressively. She also complained of nausea and has been able to eat only sparingly during the preceding 72 hours. She denied any change in bowel habits and noted no hematochezia or hematemesis. The woman's medical history was remarkable for a myocardial infarction 3 years prior to her present admission. Current medications included isosorbide, propranolol, and hydrochlorothiazide. She had had no prior operations and denied any drug allergies.

On examination, the patient's pulse was 80 beats/min, her blood pressure was 110/60 mm Hg, her respiratory rate was 24 breaths/min, and her temperature was 102° F. The patient's abdomen was distended, and marked tenderness with rebound was noted in the epigastrium. The remainder of the examination was unremarkable. Initial laboratory studies showed:

| Hb | Hct | WBC | Na | K | Cl | BUN | Cr | Amyl |
|---|---|---|---|---|---|---|---|---|
| 15 | 45 | 20,000 | 145 | 3 | 116 | 46 | 2 | 200 |

Urinalysis: specific gravity, 1.028; WBC, 0; RBC, 0; bacteria, 0; bilirubin, 0
ECG: sinus rhythm, evidence of old inferior wall MI
CXR: no active pulmonary disease, mild cardiomegaly, presence of free air under right hemidiaphragm

- *List your differential diagnosis for this patient. In addition, detail your management plan; include your plans for resuscitation, monitoring, whether or not any further diagnostic studies are needed, and the timing of operation (if necessary).*

This patient most likely has a perforated viscus. The differential diagnosis includes perforation of a gastric or duodenal ulcer, perforated diverticulum, or, possibly, a perforated colonic carcinoma. Independent of the diagnosis, the patient has signs of peritoneal irritation with

This chapter can be studied in conjunction with *Essentials of Surgical Critical Care,* edited by Jerome H. Abrams and Frank B. Cerra (St. Louis: Quality Medical Publishing, Inc., 1993), Chapters 22, 34, and *35.* Italicized number indicates the main chapter reference.

evidence of perforation on upright CXR film. Urgent operative intervention will be required after stabilization.

Aggressive resuscitation is needed to enable the patient to be brought to the operating room as soon as possible. Although her vital signs appear stable, she is known to be undergoing both diuretic and beta-blocker therapy. The history, physical examination, and initial laboratory values confirm dehydration. With this patient's cardiac history, volume resuscitation should be done judiciously. Ideally, a pulmonary artery catheter should be placed and a preoperative "tune-up" should be performed either in the SICU or in the preinduction area. With experienced personnel, these interventions will not unduly delay operative intervention. The goal of preoperative resuscitation is safer induction of general anesthesia.

ECG monitoring, nasogastric tube decompression, and urinary bladder catheterization also should be instituted. Prophylactic antibiotics should be given at least 1 hour prior to surgery. Some type of prophylaxis for deep venous thrombosis (pneumatic compression stockings or subcutaneous heparin) also should be given. No further diagnostic studies are required for this patient.

## CASE 2

You are asked to see a 66-year-old man who developed acute abdominal pain 4 days after undergoing elective three-vessel coronary artery bypass.

- *Formulate a differential diagnosis by considering the most common nonsurgical and surgical causes of acute abdominal pain in such a patient. Discuss adjunctive diagnostic tests that can be used to limit the possible diagnoses. Discuss the risk factors associated with poor prognosis in such a patient who subsequently develops an acute surgical abdomen.*

### DIFFERENTIAL DIAGNOSIS

1. *Myocardial infarction.* Serial electrocardiograms should be reviewed, and CPK-MB isoenzyme analysis should be done.

2. *Pneumonia.* CXR findings of infiltrate or changing effusion should be noted. Such findings, along with the presence of a positive sputum culture, would favor the diagnosis of pneumonia.

3. *Pancreatitis.* Elevation of the serum amylase concentration and sonographic evidence of an enlarged pancreas or peripancreatic fluid favor acute pancreatitis. If sonography cannot be performed reliably, a dynamic CT scan also would help with this diagnosis.

4. *Gastritis/peptic ulcer disease.* The presence of heme-positive nasogastric aspirate, a gastric pH $<4$, and free air under the diaphragm suggest a perforation. A gastrointestinal contrast study can be done to confirm the diagnosis, especially if nonoperative treatment of a duodenal ulcer perforation is contemplated.

5. *Decreased intestinal blood flow.* Decreased perfusion predisposes the patient to ischemic colitis, bowel infarction, and colonic perforation. Adequate cardiac output must be ensured, and any fluid and electrolyte abnormalities need to be corrected. An unexplained metabolic acidosis or rising lactate concentration should suggest mesenteric ischemia. Elevated serum phosphorous concentration is consistent with intestinal ischemia. The presence of free air suggests perforation. Visceral angiography may be necessary to diagnose bowel ischemia. *(Remember:* Do not delay operative intervention by performing unnecessary adjunctive diagnostic tests in patients who have peritoneal findings.)

6. *Acalculous cholecystitis.* An elevation of total bilirubin values suggests acalculous cholecystitis. Sonography of the right upper quadrant of the abdomen may reveal the presence of pericholecystic fluid abscess formation in the gallbladder fossa demonstrated as a thickened gallbladder wall. Nuclear studies usually are not helpful since most patients have been npo at this point in their postoperative course.

■ ■ ■

Major medical problems and postcardiopulmonary bypass complications should be considered in patients suspected of having an acute surgical abdomen after cardiac surgery. These problems and complications are associated with a high mortality rate. Cardiac operations done as emergency procedures, prolonged extracorporeal perfusion, and cardiac reoperations contribute to a poorer prognosis in patients who subsequently develop an acute surgical abdomen. In general, an aggressive, directed workup of the abdominal pain should be done while adequate resuscitation is ensured. Prompt surgical intervention should be performed when indicated.

# SECTION 6 *Endocrine System*

# CHAPTER 29

## *Endocrine Disorders*

Carol H. Wysham

### CASE 1

A 64-year-old man presented for management of deep venous thrombosis of the left leg, which had been diagnosed by outpatient venous Doppler ultrasonography. His medical history was remarkable only for atrial fibrillation, for which he was taking procainamide 1000 mg every 6 hours. On physical examination, he was noted as being a healthy obese man with a blood pressure of 160/80. His pulse was regular at 88 beats/min, and his temperature was 99.7° F. His left leg was edematous without ulceration, and he had a positive Homan's sign. The abdominal examination was unremarkable, but the stool was guaiac-positive. Admission laboratory data revealed normal electrolytes (see summary, p. 134), a hematocrit of 29.9%, WBC count of 6400/mm$^3$, erythrocyte sedimentation rate of 85, and a PTT of 48 sec. A 1:1 mix of the patient's serum with normal serum failed to correct the PTT, leading the laboratory technician to comment on the presence of "lupuslike" inhibitor. Antibody testing confirmed the presence of anticardiolipin antibody.

Procainamide, considered to be responsible for the anticardiolipin antibody, was discontinued at the request of the hematology consultant, and heparin therapy was initiated. With the exception of a low-grade fever, the patient did well until hospital day 3, when he complained of left upper quadrant abdominal pain. The examination was remarkable for moderate abdominal tenderness without guarding or rebound. The patient had normal bowel sounds.

- *What are your diagnostic considerations? How will you proceed?*

In addition to the usual causes for nontraumatic abdominal pain in a man of this age (i.e., peptic ulcer disease, pyelonephritis, intra-abdominal abscess, bowel ischemia, pancreatitis, and volvulus), the presence of anticardiolipin antibody increases the risk of venous thrombosis of the bowel, liver, and kidneys. In addition, anticoagulation would put this patient at considerable

This chapter can be studied in conjunction with *Essentials of Surgical Critical Care*, edited by Jerome H. Abrams and Frank B. Cerra (St. Louis: Quality Medical Publishing, Inc., 1993), Chapters 5, 9, 12, 30, 31, *38*, and 44. Italicized number indicates the main chapter reference.

risk for bleeding into the GI tract, spleen, retroperitoneum, and adrenal gland. An abdominal film, WBC count, hematocrit, PT, PTT, urinalysis, and stool for occult blood should be obtained.

> The abdominal flat plate showed nonspecific gas pattern without free air or ileus. Urinalysis was negative for blood or WBCs, and the stool was hemoccult-negative. The WBC count was 8000 with a left shift, and the hematocrit was 29.2.
>
> ▪ *How would you proceed?*

It is obvious that serial abdominal examination is warranted. However, in an anticoagulated patient, unexplained abdominal pain should be investigated further, ideally with an abdominal CT scan, to evaluate for intra-abdominal or retroperitonal hemorrhage. Special attention should be directed to the adrenal gland.

> Since the abdominal pain appeared to be resolving, no further investigation was pursued. On hospital day 7, the patient was noted to have a drop in blood pressure to 95/60, which returned to 130/80 after a 500 ml flush of normal saline.
>
> ▪ *How would you proceed?*

In the anticoagulated patient, a drop in blood pressure should be considered evidence for a bleed until proven otherwise. A hematocrit and WBC count should be obtained. With the previous history of unexplained abdominal pain, an abdominal CT scan is warranted.

> The hematocrit was 30.3%, and the WBC count was 8800/mm$^3$. The next morning, the patient became dyspneic with a temperature of 103° F and blood pressure of 80/40.
>
> ▪ *What would you do at this point?*

Although a pulmonary embolus is unlikely in a patient who is anticoagulated, this patient is at high risk of thromboembolic phenomena because of the anticardiolipin antibody. A pulmonary embolus must be excluded. Additional considerations include pneumonia, sepsis, myocardial infarction, and pericarditis. Finally, in the absence of an obvious cause, adrenal insufficiency should be ruled out in a hypotensive patient who is anticoagulated. A ventilation/perfusion (V/Q) scan (or pulmonary angiography), CXR, WBC count, cosyntropin stimulation test, ECG, and echocardiogram should be obtained.

> A V/Q scan showed low probability for pulmonary embolus, the ECG showed atrial fibrillation without acute ST-segment and T-wave changes. The echocardiogram was negative for pericardial fluid. The WBC count was 12,000 with a left shift. The patient was transferred to the ICU. His blood pressure failed to respond to fluid resuscitation and administration of dopamine. On hemodynamic monitoring, the patient's cardiac output was 10, and systemic vascular resistance was 456. Blood cultures were drawn and broad-spectrum antibiotics were started for the presumptive diagnosis of sepsis. One of four blood culture bottles was later found to be positive for *Staphylococcus aureus*. The patient continued to be hypotensive for the next 36 hours, when the possibility of adrenal insufficiency was raised. A cosyntropin stimulation test was performed, followed by the intravenous administration of 100 mg of hydrocortisone. The patient's blood pressure and hemodynamic values improved dramatically within 6 hours, and the use of dopamine was discontinued. The basal cortisol was 1.5 μg/dl and was not stimulated by the administration of cosyntropin. An abdominal CT scan revealed marked enlargement of the right adrenal gland, whereas the left adrenal was not visualized. The remainder of the patient's hospital course was uneventful. He was discharged

in stable condition, and therapy was continued with hydrocortisone (20 mg in the morning and 20 mg in the evening), coumadin, and digoxin.

*Summary of Hospital Course*

| Date | Temp (° F) | BP (mm Hg) | Hct (%) | Plt ($\times 10^3$)/mm$^3$ | WBC ($\times 10^3$)/Eos | Na (mEq/L) | K (mEq/L) | BUN (mg/dl) |
|---|---|---|---|---|---|---|---|---|
| 9/5 | 99.1 | 160/80 | 29.9 | 215 | 6.4/0 | 139 | 4.1 | 10 |
| 9/6 | 100.8 | 130/80 | 27.3 | 125 | 5.5/0 | | | |
| 9/8 | 101.6 | 116/58 | 29.2 | 131 | 8.0/0 | | | |
| 9/9 | 100.2 | 142/64 | 30.2 | 131 | 9.3/0 | 138 | 4.2 | 20 |
| 9/10 | 101.6 | 152/60 | 30.0 | 105 | 8.8/88 | 137 | 4.1 | 25 |
| 9/11 | 100.6 | 95/60 | 30.3 | 96 | 9.8/98 | 135 | 3.6 | 24 |
| 9/12 | 103.0 | 80/40 | 28.1 | 137 | 12.0/120 | 131 | 4.1 | 54 |
| 9/13 | 102.2 | 85/45 | 29.3 | 141 | 11.0/173 | 139 | 4.0 | |
| 9/14 | 98.2 | 130/70 | 30.0 | 160 | 8.2/0 | 141 | 3.8 | 41 |

The development of adrenal insufficiency from thrombosis or hemorrhage in patients with the anticardiolipin antibody syndrome has been reported in at least 20 cases. Such patients frequently develop vascular thromboses, often requiring therapeutic anticoagulation. In addition to the presence of the anticardiolipin antibody, this patient was therapeutically anticoagulated with heparin, which put him at additional risk for adrenal hemorrhage. Several clinical clues suggest the development of adrenal hemorrhage/thrombosis in this case. The development of abdominal pain on 9/8 is very suggestive of this condition. Indeed, adrenal insufficiency should be routinely considered when unexplained abdominal pain occurs in a patient with a bleeding diathesis. An abdominal CT scan done at this time would have confirmed the diagnosis, allowing for the performance of biochemical testing and the initiation of glucocorticoid treatment prior to the development of vascular collapse, which carries a very high mortality. In light of this patient's very low cortisol concentrations, his abdominal CT findings were interpreted as consistent with hemorrhage of the right adrenal gland and possible thrombosis of the left adrenal gland. The characteristic electrolyte changes (hyponatremia and hyperkalemia) were absent in this case, as frequently occurs in adrenal hemorrhage, in which fluid and electrolytes are managed carefully. However, there was a progressive rise in the BUN. Finally, the appearance of significant numbers of eosinophils on 9/11, at a time when the patient was severely ill, is a subtle finding that points to the presence of adrenal insufficiency.

The management of adrenal crisis should include: (1) appropriate hemodynamic support with normal saline (usually as 5% dextrose in normal saline to prevent hypoglycemia) and pressors, (2) hydrocortisone 100 mg IV every 8 hours, and (3) treatment of underlying disease.

The rapid normalization of blood pressure and temperature after glucocorticoid therapy that was seen in this patient is typical for patients with adrenal crisis.

## CASE 2

A 64-year-old man who was not wearing a seatbelt was a driver involved in a motor vehicle accident. He suffered multiple rib fractures, pneumothorax, and left acetabular fracture. Chest tubes were placed, and the patient did well until hospital day 9, when he developed severe dyspnea and hypotension with blood pressure of 54/40. He was intubated and his blood pressure was supported with a dopamine infusion. A diagnosis of massive pulmonary embolus was made at angiography. The patient was treated with recombinant tissue plasminogen activator, followed by heparin infusion. He subsequently developed staphylococcal sepsis and massive bleeding from his chest tubes, requiring ligation of several intercostal arteries. Despite the administration of dopamine, dobutamine, epinephrine, and amrinone, the patient's systolic blood pressure remained below 90 mm Hg for 48 hours, resulting in the development of acute renal failure. On hospital day 18, hemodialysis was begun. The patient's subsequent course was complicated by bacterial and fungal septicemia, hypotension requiring long-term dopamine therapy, pericardial tamponade, adult respiratory distress syndrome, hypermetabolism, coma, and recurrent episodes of acute renal failure, necessitating intermittent hemodialysis for 2 months. On hospital day 65, thyroid function tests were ordered and a cosyntropin stimulation test was performed. The following results were noted:

$T_4$RIA ($T_4$ radioimmunoassay): <1.0 μg/dl
THBR (thyroid hormone-binding ratio): 1.81
FTI (free thyroxine index): <1.8
$T_3$RIA ($T_3$ radioimmunoassay): 52 ng/dl
TSH (thyroid-stimulating hormone): 3.93 μU/ml
Basal cortisol: 26.7 μg/dl
60 min after cosyntropin: 24.8 μg/dl

An endocrinologic consultation was obtained, and the diagnosis of hypothyroidism was made. Whether the condition was caused by primary thyroid dysfunction or associated with prolonged dopamine infusion was unclear. Adrenal function was considered to be adequate. Levothyroxine 100 μg was given intravenously and continued on a daily basis. Two days later, the patient was alert. Over the next week, his blood pressure stabilized and renal function improved. The dopamine infusion and dialysis were discontinued. After 11 days of levothyroxine therapy, the patient was noted to be "vastly improved." He was extubated and, after prolonged rehabilitation, was discharged 3 months after admission.

This case includes no historical features to suggest preexisting hypothyroidism. Therefore thyroid function testing was not performed on admission. It is difficult to say, even in retrospect, when this patient developed hypothyroidism. At no time during his course did he demonstrate any of the classic features of hypothyroidism, including hypothermia, bradycardia, and dry skin. Hyponatremia and impaired free water excretion were obscured by renal failure. The first clue to the possibility of superimposed hypothyroidism was the patient's altered mental status. However, at the time this was easily explained by the multitude of systemic insults. The development of pericardial effusion is common in severe hypothyroidism, but pericardial tamponade occurs rarely. When fluid is obtained, it is generally transudative. An increased susceptibility to sepsis has been reported in hypothyroid patients. In this patient the diagnosis of hypothyroidism was considered only after he failed to respond to the usual therapeutic measures.

The thyroid function tests might have been interpreted as representative of those associated with nonthyroidal illness. However, in such patients, the free thyroxine index is rarely <2. More likely, the unmeasurable $T_4$ level was caused by preexisting primary hypothyroidism, with blunting of the usual TSH elevation by prolonged dopamine infusion. Alternatively, the use of dopamine therapy extending over several weeks may have suppressed TSH secretion to a sufficient degree to decrease serum $T_4$ levels. Since the serum half-life of thyroxine is 7 days, 2 to 3 weeks of dopamine therapy probably would be necessary to alter thyroxine levels to this extent.

When faced with a patient in whom myxedema coma appears to be likely, an emergency endocrinology consultation is warranted. If unavailable, blood for $T_4$, THBR, and TSH should be obtained, and therapy should be instituted without delay. An intravenous dose of 100 to 200 μg of levothyroxine and 25 μg of oral triiodothyronine should be given, followed by a daily dose of 50 to 100 μg of levothyroxine. Triiodothyronine at a dose of 25 to 50 μg bid is continued until patient's clinical status has improved, generally 2 to 4 days.

Finally, the course of improvement in this patient's clinical condition after levothyroxine therapy is consistent with that seen in the treatment of myxedema coma, in which the majority of patients experience improvement in mental status within 36 hours of initiation of treatment.

# CHAPTER 30

# *Divalent Ions*

John E. Mazuski

## CASE 1

A 46-year-old man was brought to the hospital after being stabbed in the abdomen. He had been hospitalized frequently for acute alcoholic intoxication in the past. On arrival, the patient was hypotensive and tachycardic and had an obvious hemoperitoneum. The patient received volume resuscitation and was quickly taken to the operating room, where exploratory laparotomy revealed profusely bleeding wounds to the right lobe of the liver, the inferior vena cava, and the right renal vein, as well as a duodenal laceration. These wounds were repaired, during which time the patient required 18 units of packed RBCs, along with approximately 10 L of crystalloid. During surgery, the calcium concentration was checked and noted to be 6.4 mg/dl; the patient then received 2 g of calcium gluconate intraoperatively. After surgery, the patient was taken directly to the SICU, where he was noted to have a temperature of 33.8° C (92.8° F), blood pressure of 90/60, and a pulse rate of 120, with frequent premature ventricular contractions (PVCs). Urine output had been 75 ml over the preceding hour. Further fluid resuscitation of this patient was undertaken after placement of a Swan-Ganz catheter and will not be discussed here. Laboratory studies that were obtained on the patient's arrival in the SICU were reported as follows: total calcium, 5.9 mg/dl; ionized calcium, 2.6 mg/dl; magnesium, 1.2 mg/dl; and phosphorus, 1.5 mg/dl.

- *What are the possible etiologic factors for these abnormalities? What treatment should be undertaken?*

This patient manifests abnormalities of all divalent ions. Several factors may contribute to the abnormalities in this patient. In part, the hypocalcemia may be caused by the complexing of calcium by citrate administered with the blood transfusions. Although citrate is normally metabolized rapidly, hypothermia and hypovolemic shock may inhibit this metabolism. In addition, hypovolemic shock may have allowed ionized calcium to be lost into the intracellular space. The patient's social history also puts him at risk for significant malnutrition, and he may have had preexisting hypocalcemia. Hypoalbuminemia associated with massive volume replacement may be important in the decreased total serum calcium concentrations, but this would not affect the ionized calcium levels.

The abnormal serum phosphorus may be a dilutional effect from massive volume replacement, but a preexisting phosphate deficiency is likely in this alcoholic patient. Similar factors may play a role in the serum magnesium abnormality.

---

This chapter can be studied in conjunction with *Essentials of Surgical Critical Care,* edited by Jerome H. Abrams and Frank B. Cerra (St. Louis: Quality Medical Publishing, Inc., 1993), Chapters 5 and *39*. Italicized number indicates the main chapter reference.

Although the abnormalities of ionized calcium and phosphorus may be transient, replacement of these divalent ions should be undertaken since chronic deficiencies are likely. The patient has PVCs, which could be exacerbated by hypomagnesemia, and magnesium also should be replaced.

> The patient received 2 g of magnesium sulfate and 1 g of calcium gluconate in the first 2 hours after his arrival in the SICU. He also received 5 mmol of phosphate, administered as a potassium salt over 3 hours, 1 hour after completion of the calcium infusion. Repeat laboratory values were then obtained. They showed: total calcium, 6.2 mg/dl; ionized calcium, 3.4 mg/dl; magnesium, 1.4 mg/dl; phosphorus, 2.4 mg/dl; and albumin, 2.1 mg/dl. The patient was continued on magnesium sulfate replacement therapy of 1 g every 6 hours. Two days later, the following values were obtained: total calcium, 7.1 mg/dl; ionized calcium, 4.1 mg/dl; magnesium, 1.8 mg/dl; phosphorus, 2.4 mg/dl; and albumin, 2.2 mg/dl. This patient was then started on total parenteral nutrition, which contained 10 mmol of calcium, 10 mEq of magnesium, and 15 mmol of phosphate per day. Laboratory values obtained the next morning showed: total calcium, 7.3 mg/dl; ionized calcium, 4.3 mg/dl; magnesium, 1.5 mg/dl; phosphorus, 1.3 mg/dl; and albumin, 2.2 mg/dl.
>
> ▪ *What factors contributed to these new abnormalities?*

This patient probably had severe preexisting deficits in total body stores of both magnesium and phosphorus. Usually 5 to 7 days are needed to replete these stores, and it is unlikely that full replacement had been achieved after 3 days of therapy. These deficits became more apparent because the patient was subjected to glucose loading, which caused release of insulin and shifting of phosphorus and magnesium intracellularly. Supplementation of both magnesium and phosphorus should be continued for several days more until these stores are adequately repleted. Thus, in addition to sufficient amounts of magnesium and phosphate to meet daily maintenance requirements, supplemental amounts of these agents, either added directly to the TPN solution or administered separately, are needed.

The normal ionized serum calcium indicates that the low total serum calcium is most likely caused by hypoalbuminemia. Thus administration of additional calcium beyond maintenance requirements is not needed.

## CASE 2

> A 66-year-old woman was admitted to the hospital because of dehydration following several days of increasing lethargy and vomiting. She had a history of metastatic breast cancer, for which she was receiving tamoxifen, and a history of hypertension, for which she was receiving hydrochlorothiazide. On examination, the patient was moaning and unable to give any coherent answers. Blood pressure was 140/60 with a pulse rate of 68 beats/min in the supine position. These values changed to a blood pressure of 90/50 with a pulse rate of 76 when the patient was put in the sitting position. Physical examination also was remarkable for dry mucous membranes and markedly diminished deep tendon reflexes. Laboratory examination showed these values: sodium, 138 mEq/L; potassium, 4.2 mEq/L; chloride, 96 mEq/L; carbon dioxide, 26 mEq/L; urea nitrogen, 70 mg/dl; creatinine, 2.1 mg/dl; calcium, 15.2 mg/dl; phosphorus, 4.5 mg/dl; and magnesium, 2.3 mg/dl.
>
> ▪ *What are the causes of this patient's hypercalcemia? What therapy should be instituted?*

This patient most likely has hypercalcemia resulting from malignancy, which has been exacerbated by dehydration and the use of a thyazide diuretic. Initial therapy for this patient should be rehydration and forced diuresis.

The patient was given 2 L of saline over the following 2 hours. Urine output was only 15 ml during that period. To guide resuscitation of this patient, a Swan-Ganz catheter was placed. The initial values included a central venous pressure of 4 and a pulmonary capillary wedge pressure (PCWP) of 5 mm Hg. Hydration was continued at a rate of 500 ml/hr while these measurements were followed. After another 2 hours, the PCWP had increased to 15 mm Hg, but the patient's urine output was only 35 ml over those 2 hours. Repeat serum calcium at this time was 14.3 mg/dl. Saline administration was continued at a rate of 200 ml/hr and 20 mg of furosemide was administered. Shortly thereafter a brisk diuresis ensued and continued over the next 6 hours with this therapy. The serum calcium concentration was again measured and was found to be 11.6 mg/dl. The patient was able to answer coherently, although she was still somewhat lethargic. Tendon reflexes now could be elicited. Over the next 48 hours the patient's overall condition stabilized, and intravenous fluid therapy was discontinued. However, serum calcium remained in the range of 11 to 12 mg/dl.

- *What additional therapy might be considered at this point?*

Although this patient has ongoing hypercalcemia, additional therapy for malignancy-induced hypercalcemia is a matter of debate. Since her initial episode of altered mental status and vomiting could have been caused by hypercalcemia, such therapy could be considered. Medications that could be used include mithramycin, calcitonin, corticosteroids, and diphosphonates, all of which inhibit reabsorption of bone. In any case, the patient should be warned against future use of thyazide diuretics, which promote calcium reabsorption and hypercalcemia. If fluid retention is a problem, a loop diuretic would be preferable.

# PART FOUR

# *SYSTEMIC DYSFUNCTION*

# CHAPTER 31

# *Intra-abdominal Infection*

Ori D. Rotstein • Richard L. Simmons

## CASE 1

A 75-year-old woman was reviewed with a 5-year history of chronic diarrhea associated with crampy abdominal pain and bloating. Investigations revealed clear evidence of a partial distal small bowel obstruction, probably related to Crohn's disease. She was admitted to the hospital for ileocecal resection to manage the Crohn's disease.

Preoperatively, the patient received Go-Lytely and an antibiotic preparation of oral neomycin plus erythromycin. Immediately prior to her operation, she received intravenous injection with gentamicin 80 mg and metronidazole 500 mg. The patient underwent an uncomplicated ileocecal resection with a primary anastomosis performed with staplers. Both gross and microscopic pathology reports indicated the presence of ileocecal Crohn's disease. The resection margins were free of residual Crohn's disease.

Postoperatively, the patient initially did well. On day 5, she began developing febrile episodes with rectal temperatures rising as high as 38.7° C (101.5° F). Clinical examination revealed a tender fullness on the right side of the abdomen. The patient's leukocyte count was elevated to 16,000 cells/mm$^3$. Fig. 31-1 illustrates the abdominal CT scan of this patient. Clear evidence of an abscess on the right side of the abdomen is noted (Fig. 31-1, *A*). This abscess was drained percutaneously (Fig. 31-1, *B*), and the patient was started on antibiotic therapy, which consisted of imipenem/cilastatin, 500 mg q 6 hr. The patient's fever and leukocytosis rapidly subsided, and her general state of well-being improved. On day 7, following insertion of the percutaneous catheter, a sinogram was performed. Fig. 31-2 illustrates a small connection to the GI tract, which indicates an enterocutaneous fistula. The antibiotics were discontinued, and the patient was discharged to home with the drainage tube in place. There was minimal drainage from the tube itself.

Two weeks following discharge from the hospital, a sinogram revealed no continued connection to the small bowel, and the catheter was removed. The patient was seen in follow-up 1 month following discharge from the hospital. She appeared well and had an excellent appetite.

This woman developed a localized postoperative abscess as a result of an anastomotic breakdown. The abscess was effectively treated with percutaneous drainage and broad-spectrum antimicrobial therapy. The percutaneous drain not only successfully treated the abscess but also permitted healing of the enterocutaneous fistula.

---

This chapter can be studied in conjunction with *Essentials of Surgical Critical Care,* edited by Jerome H. Abrams and Frank B. Cerra (St. Louis: Quality Medical Publishing, Inc., 1993), Chapter 40.

A B

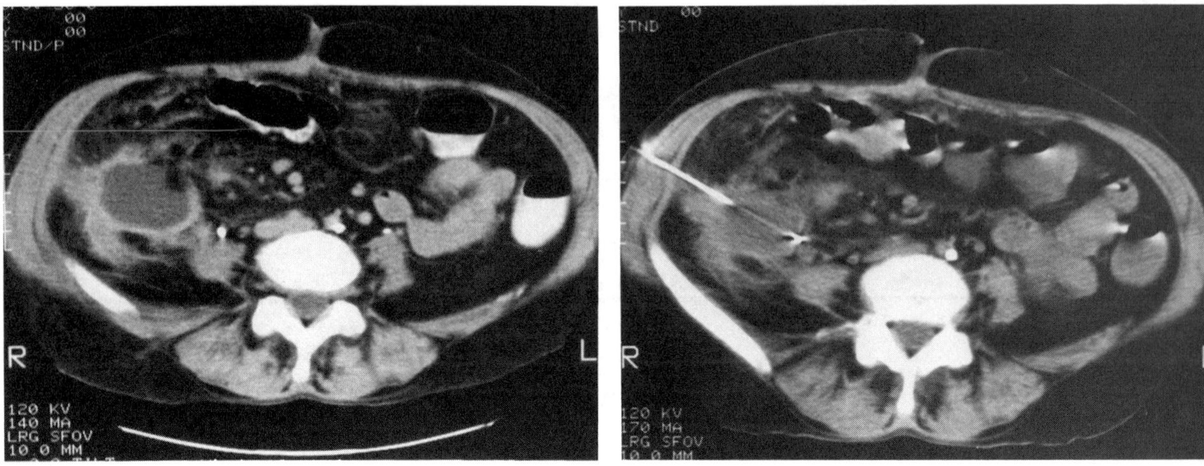


FIG 31-1

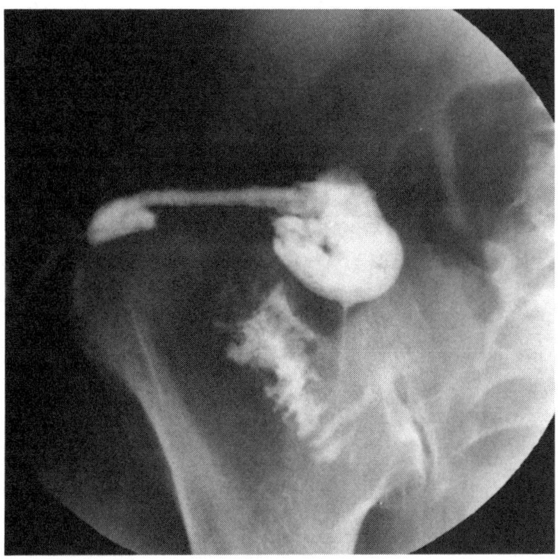

FIG 31-2

In the judgment of the patient's surgeon, percutaneous drainage was of lower risk than reexploration and it offered sufficient potential for adequately treating the abscess. Percutaneous therapy was initiated with the plan of doing reexploration if clear clinical improvement did not occur rapidly.

## CASE 2

A 22-year-old man presented to the emergency department with an 18-hour history of crampy periumbilical pain that progressed into the right lower quadrant. Associated fever, nausea, and vomiting were present. Clinical examination revealed an ill young man with a temperature of 38.5° C (101.5° F) and right lower quadrant peritoneal signs. The leukocyte count was 18,500 $mm^3$. The urinalysis was negative, and abdominal x-ray films were not helpful.

The patient was taken to the operating room following a 2 L fluid resuscitation with crystalloid and a single dose of cefotetan, 1 g IV. A laparotomy was performed through a McBurney's incision. The appendix was found to be perforated at its base, and some purulent fluid was present in the right lower quadrant. The appendix was removed, and lavage of the right lower quadrant was done with warm saline solution until all purulent material had been evacuated. The peritoneum and the external oblique aponeurosis were closed. The skin and subcutaneous tissues were left open, but Prolene sutures were left in place untied for delayed closure.

Postoperatively, the patient made a rapid recovery. By day 4, he was feeling well and tolerating a full diet. He was afebrile and had a normal leukocyte count for 48 hours. The wound surface appeared to be showing initial evidence of granulation. Antibiotics were discontinued, the wound was closed, and the patient was discharged to home on day 4.

This case demonstrates the principles of management of peritonitis: fluid resuscitation, broad-spectrum antibiotic therapy, and appropriate surgical intervention. Postoperatively, this patient's rapid clinical response allowed early discontinuation of antibiotics and discharge from the hospital.

# CHAPTER 32

# *Burns, Electrical Injury, and Hypothermia and Frostbite*

David H. Ahrenholz • Lynn D. Solem

## CASE 1

A 32-year-old man was rescued from an apartment fire after he fell asleep on the couch with a lighted cigarette. The victim was comatose but breathing spontaneously. The paramedics started 100% oxygen by nonrebreathing mask and Ringer's lactate via a 16-gauge catheter in the antecubital fossa. All clothing and jewelry were removed. The patient was noted to have deep burns of the head, neck, trunk, and both upper extremities, sparing only the axillae. The patient was covered with a clean sheet and transported to the emergency room.

The patient should be quickly evaluated as with any other trauma patient—ABC. The patient is spontaneously breathing at present, but in view of the inhalation injury he will need endotracheal intubation and assisted ventilation (100% oxygen until the carbon monoxide has cleared). The patient's other vital signs are stable. In addition to the endotracheal tube, the patient needs a Foley catheter for monitoring of urine output, a nasogastric tube to decompress the stomach, and fluid resuscitation with Ringer's lactate solution.

The burn size initially can be estimated with the "rule of nines":

| Location | Burn (%) |
|---|---|
| Head and neck | 9 |
| Anterior trunk | 18 |
| Posterior trunk | 18 |
| Left arm | 9 |
| Right arm | 9 |
| APPROXIMATE TOTAL | 63 |

The Parkland formula is used with an estimated weight of 70 kg (4 ml/kg/% burn): $4 \times 70 \times 63 = 17{,}640$ ml. Half the volume, or approximately 9 L, is given in the first 8 hours; the other half is given in the following 16 hours. The rate will be ~1100 ml/hr for the first 8 hours and may be adjusted for urine output (minimum of 30 ml/hr), pulse <120, and blood pressure >100 mm Hg.

This chapter can be studied in conjunction with *Essentials of Surgical Critical Care,* edited by Jerome H. Abrams and Frank B. Cerra (St. Louis: Quality Medical Publishing, Inc., 1993), Chapters 5 and *42*. Italicized number indicates the main chapter reference.

## CASE 2

The patient was a 78-year-old woman who was found lying on the floor of her apartment. She had shallow respirations at a rate of 8/min, a thready femoral pulse, and a sinus bradycardia of 40. She responded to deep pain by moaning and moved her left side weakly. The paramedics started oxygen by mask, Ringer's lactate by a 16-gauge catheter in the antecubital vein, and transported the patient to the emergency department.

On arrival at the emergency department, the patient's clothing was removed, and a rapid survey revealed an adequate airway but inadequate air exchange. The patient was intubated in a blind fashion via the nasotracheal route because the status of the cervical spine was unknown. The patient's vital signs were: pulse, 36; blood pressure, 60 systolic; and core temperature, 82° F (28° C). The patient was ventilated with heated (40° C) and humidified 100% oxygen.

Warmed saline was rapidly infused while electrolytes and blood gases were checked. A Foley catheter also was placed. The patient had two peritoneal lavage catheters placed percutaneously (directed into the peritoneal gutters), and rapid lavage was started. Non–potassium-containing dialysate was warmed in the microwave oven to 104° to 108° F (40° to 42° C) and rapidly infused into one of the lavage catheters, with the other catheter used as a drainage catheter. During this process the patient underwent computed tomography of the head, which showed an acute subdural hematoma.

# CHAPTER 33

# *Anaphylaxis*

Paul Druck

## CASE 1

An 18-year-old man was admitted to the emergency department with gunshot wounds of the left chest and left upper quadrant of the abdomen. After receiving 800 ml of crystalloid solution en route, the patient's blood pressure was 105/60 and his pulse was 110. Physical examination revealed abdominal tenderness and guarding; no other injuries were noted. A left chest tube was inserted and drained 350 ml of blood. CXR film demonstrated the chest tube in appropriate position, with no residual hemothorax or pneumothorax. A decision was made to perform prompt exploratory laparotomy, and the patient received 1 g of a first-generation cephalosporin. A nasogastric tube and a Foley catheter were inserted. Gross hematuria was noted and a "one-shot" intravenous pyelogram was obtained quickly in the emergency department. Just prior to transport to the operating room, the patient complained of shortness of breath and a "lump in the throat." His blood pressure was noted as 90/50; pulse, 120; and a total of 1800 ml of crystalloid had been given. Auscultation of the chest revealed noisy respirations bilaterally, with possible wheezing. The chest tube had not drained a significant amount of blood since the initial drainage.

- *What is your evaluation?*

In a trauma patient, hypotension always should raise the concern of ongoing blood loss, and respiratory distress should suggest unrecognized or untreated thoracic or cervical injuries. However, other pathologic conditions are possible in trauma patients, and the development of hypotension, respiratory distress, and symptoms referable to the pharynx or the upper airway are highly suggestive of anaphylaxis, particularly after administration of pharmaceuticals capable of causing such a reaction. Indeed, beta-lactam antibiotics and iodinated radiocontrast material together account for the overwhelming majority of such reactions among hospitalized patients. Their potential for causing reactions should be borne in mind *whenever* they are used.

Two units of type O-negative packed RBCs were started, a repeat CXR film and an arterial blood gas study were obtained, and the chest tube was stripped and noted to be patent. The results of the ABG study were: pH, 7.43; $P_{CO_2}$, 30; and $P_{O_2}$, 72. The CXR film showed clear lung fields bilaterally, no hemothorax or pneumothorax, and no mediastinal shift. The patient's blood pressure remained 90/50, and he was taken to the operating room expeditiously. On arrival in the operating room, he demonstrated stridor and agitation.

- *How would you manage the patient at this time?*

---

This chapter can be studied in conjunction with *Essentials of Surgical Critical Care,* edited by Jerome H. Abrams and Frank B. Cerra (St. Louis: Quality Medical Publishing, Inc., 1993), Chapters 5, 11, 12, 24, 25, 27, and *43*. Italicized number indicates the main chapter reference.

The patient has upper airway obstruction. Regardless of the cause, establishing a secure, patent airway is an urgent priority. In fact, it would have been appropriate to do this in the emergency department *prior to transport* because (1) the patient was hemodynamically unstable with respiratory distress, and (2) anaphylaxis with impending upper airway obstruction should have been considered.

The patient's hypotension was treated with fluids and blood products appropriate for hemorrhage and initially suitable for anaphylasis. However, if the patient's blood pressure fails to respond adequately and anaphylaxis is still not considered, the need for beta-agonists or pressors may go unrecognized.

Endotracheal intubation was attempted in the operating room, but it was impossible because of the patient's severe agitation and marked glottic edema. A cricothyroidotomy was performed promptly, and the patient was ventilated and oxygenated. Noting bilateral wheezing, resistance to manual ventilation, glottic edema, and the patient's blood pressure, which had fallen to 80/50 as his agitation subsided, the anesthesiologist suggested the possibility of anaphylaxis and was informed that the patient had received a cephalosporin antibiotic and iodinated radiocontrast material. Epinephrine 1:100,000 10 ml IV, benadryl 50 mg IV, and hydrocortisone 100 mg IV were administered. These agents produced decreased wheezing and airway pressures and increased blood pressure. Exploratory laparotomy, nephrectomy, and colostomy were performed. During these procedures, the patient required epinephrine one more time for wheezing, and an aminophylline drip was prepared but not required. In the recovery room, the patient's vital signs were stable, his breath sounds were clear, and arterial blood gases on mechanical ventilation were adequate without excessive airway pressures.

- *How would you monitor and manage the patient's subsequent respiratory and cardiovascular care?*

The clinical syndrome and response to epinephrine strongly suggest anaphylaxis. The priority now is preventing or, if necessary, treating recurrent symptoms. The patient should be monitored in an SICU for at least 24 hours and receive full-dose parenteral hydrocortisone (100 to 200 mg IV, q 4 to 6 hr) for 24 hours, followed by rapid tapering if no symptoms recur. Extubation may be performed when direct laryngoscopy demonstrates resolution of glottic edema. The responsible agent should be identified, if possible, by review of the medication record and by obtaining relevant history from the patient or his family. All potentially responsible agents should be avoided. If a potentially cross-reacting antibiotic is strongly indicated in the postoperative period, preliminary scratch-test sensitivity should be determined, preferably in consultation with an immunologist. The patient should be informed of the episode and instructed about suitable precautions in the future.

## CASE 2

You were called to see a patient in the SICU because of increasing airway pressures (peak pressure, 55 cm $H_2O$; plateau pressure, 25 cm $H_2O$), and reduced oxyhemoglobin saturation by pulse oximetry ($O_2$ saturation, 88% on an $F_{IO_2}$ of 0.3). One day earlier the patient had undergone emergency repair of a leaking abdominal aortic aneurysm and was expected to be extubated soon. On morning rounds, he was noted to be febrile to 101° F, had significant wound erythema, and penicillin G 2 million units IV q 6 hr was ordered. The patient had received a single preoperative dose of a first-generation cephalosporin antibiotic. A Swan-

Ganz catheter and arterial line were in place. The patient's blood pressure was 105/65, pulse was 110, and pulmonary artery pressure was 42/22.

- *What is your evaluation?*

The differential diagnosis includes ventilator malfunction, endotracheal tube occlusion, bronchospasm, pneumothorax, pulmonary edema associated with fluid overload or left ventricular failure, pulmonary embolus, and drug reaction. Adult respiratory distress syndrome would not be expected to develop precipitously. Additional history should be obtained while the differential diagnosis is being addressed and acute problems are being treated. The most immediately life-threatening problems are ventilator malfunction, endotracheal tube occlusion, and tension pneumothorax, and these should be addressed first. In addition, the patient's blood pressure is below normal with a widened pulse pressure and tachycardia. Normal or elevated blood pressure would be expected with isolated respiratory distress.

The ventilator was disconnected and evaluated while the patient was being manually ventilated with 100% oxygen. The endotracheal tube was suctioned and found to be free of kinks and secretions. Oxygen saturation had risen to 92%. On auscultation of the chest, bilaterally equal but decreased breath sounds and wheezes were heard. The abdomen was not distended, and there were no palpable popliteal cords or leg edema. A portable CXR examination, arterial blood gas study, 12-lead ECG, and CBC were obtained. Pulmonary capillary wedge pressure was 6 mm Hg, and 500 ml of 5% albumin solution was administered intravenously. The patient was returned to the ventilator and in-line nebulized metaproterenol was administered. The ABG study results were: pH, 7.48; $Pco_2$, 31; and $Po_2$, 72. The CXR film demonstrated clear but somewhat hyperinflated lung fields without pneumothorax. The patient's blood pressure was now 90/50, pulse was 115, and PCWP was 4 mm Hg, and persistent diffuse wheezes were noted on auscultation. The patient's medical history does not include chronic obstructive pulmonary disease, asthma, or drug or food allergies.

- *How would you proceed?*

Ventilator malfunction, upper airway occlusion, pulmonary edema associated with fluid overload or left ventricular failure, and pneumothorax have been ruled out. Further evaluation of pulmonary embolus is not possible until the patient's condition is stabilized. The improvement in oxygen saturation to adequate levels on increased supplemental oxygen does not rule out pulmonary embolus, but it argues against a massive episode. Presumptive heparinization 1 day after aortic surgery would not be appropriate. The possibilities at this point have been narrowed to bronchospasm without a history of bronchospastic disease.

The patient also has worsening hypotension associated with hypovolemia, without the abdominal distention that might be expected with intra-abdominal or retroperitoneal bleeding. Furthermore, hemorrhage would not explain the sudden, intense bronchospasm. At this point anaphylaxis should be considered, although pulmonary embolus remains a possibility. Epinephrine should be given, despite the compensatory tachycardia, and fluid resuscitation should be considered. The administration of blood products, any new medications, or particularly suspicious drugs, such as antibiotics, iodine-containing materials, opiates, and nonsteroidal analgesics, should be discontinued.

The blood pressure remained 90/50, PCWP fell to 4 mm Hg, and wheezing and elevated airway pressures persisted. An additional 500 ml of 5% albumin solution was administered, along with epinephrine 1:100,000 10 ml IV. Blood pressure rose to 130/70 and pulse to 125, and wheezing decreased. Urticaria was noticed on the anterior chest. After the initial response, blood pressure again fell. Hemodynamic values were obtained: BP, 100/55; PCWP,

8 mm Hg; CO/CI, 9/5.2; and SVR, 618 dyne · sec · cm$^{-5}$. An additional dose of epinephrine was administered plus additional colloid solution, but the response again was transient. A continuous epinephrine infusion was begun at 1 μg/min, with a favorable pressure response, but pulse rate rose to 130, and anterolateral ST-segment depressions were seen.

- *How would you proceed?*

If epinephrine, because of its beta-agonist properties, produces unacceptable tachycardia or dysrhythmias or myocardial ischemia, an alpha-agonist may be substituted to treat hypotension refractory to optimization of filling pressures. Because of potentially intense vasoconstriction with hypertension, excessive cardiac afterload, and visceral ischemia, the dosage of an alpha-agonist should be carefully titrated to produce the minimal acceptable blood pressure. Urine output, peripheral perfusion, and ECG should be closely monitored. Continued bronchospasm may be treated with aminophylline or inhaled bronchodilators.

The patient's PCWP was maintained at 16 mm Hg, blood pressure was titrated to 100/70 with norepinephrine, and bronchospasm was controlled with albuterol and ipratropium bromide. Signs of myocardial ischemia resolved, and weaning from the norepinephrine infusion was done slowly over the ensuing hour.

- *What further management would you recommend?*

This patient's clinical course is consistent with anaphylaxis. The most likely offending agent is the penicillin administered shortly before the onset of symptoms. Hydrocortisone 100 to 200 mg IV q 4 to 6 hr for 24 hours, followed by rapid tapering if no symptoms recur, is indicated to prevent recurrence. A follow-up CXR examination to rule out pneumothorax secondary to barotrauma and cardiac enzyme determinations to rule out myocardial infarction should be obtained. As the patient's vascular tone returns to normal, sudden fluid overload is possible, and filling pressures should be carefully monitored until the additional fluid load, some of which will be extravascular, is mobilized and diuresed. All beta-lactam antibiotics should be avoided. The episode should be documented carefully and related to the patient when appropriate.

# CHAPTER 34

## *Disorders of Coagulation*

Kathleen V. Watson • Gregory M. Vercellotti

### CASE 1

A 55-year-old woman was admitted to the SICU following coronary artery bypass graft surgery for a 95% occlusion of the proximal left coronary artery. Her medical history was significant for coronary artery disease, alcohol abuse, and cigarette smoking.

The patient had been admitted to the medical intensive care unit 3 days earlier with unstable angina. Initially she was managed with diltiazem, atenolol, nitroglycerin infusion, and aspirin. Twelve hours after admission, the patient underwent emergency coronary angiography, which revealed complete occlusion of the proximal left coronary artery. Percutaneous transluminal angioplasty (PCTA) was performed, and repeat angiography in the catheterization laboratory showed 80% perfusion. Forty-eight hours later, the patient experienced recurrent angina; the ECG showed acute anterior myocardial ischemia. The patient was taken to the operating room for emergency coronary artery bypass. Cardiopulmonary bypass (CPB) lasted for 75 minutes without complications. Routine heparinization was reversed with protamine following CPB. Laboratory studies were shown to be:

Preoperative: Normal PT, PTT, and TT
  Hemoglobin 12.5 g/dl, WBC 5800/mm$^3$, platelets 180,000/mm$^3$
Postoperative:
  6 hours: PT, PTT 1 sec prolonged
    TT 19 sec (normal 13-18)
    Hemoglobin 13 g/dl
    Platelets 108,000/mm$^3$
  12 hours: Same, except platelets 120,000/mm$^3$
    TT 19.5 sec

- *The SICU nurse pages you after the 12-hour laboratory results have been received to request platelet transfusions. What are your considerations and recommendations at this time?*

You would first ask the nurse for vital signs, current medications, and the clinical status of the patient. The nurse informs you that the arterial line blood pressure is 100/76, pulse is 100 in normal sinus rhythm, ventilatory status is stable, and temperature is 100° F. The patient has no evidence of bleeding from the thoracotomy site, endotracheal tube, venipuncture, or arterial puncture sites. Nasogastric fluid and catheterized urine are negative for blood. No purpura are present.

---

This chapter can be studied in conjunction with *Essentials of Surgical Critical Care,* edited by Jerome H. Abrams and Frank B. Cerra (St. Louis: Quality Medical Publishing, Inc., 1993), Chapter 44.

No evidence of generalized or localized bleeding has been found in the patient. Following CPB, it is common for patients to have mild abnormalities of PT and PTT that are caused by hemodilution with banked blood products. In addition, because of the patient's history of alcoholism, there may be preexisting vitamin-K deficiency on an ongoing basis. Alcoholic liver disease would predispose this patient to other acquired hemostatic abnormalities; it is necessary to remain alert for signs of such abnormalities. The most likely explanation for the prolonged TT is heparin contamination from the arterial line (depending on the concentration, such contamination also would prolong PT and PTT). Other considerations include decreased or abnormal fibrinogen as a consequence of compromised liver function, consumption, and sepsis. The thrombocytopenia is most likely the result of consumption during CPB, although other possibilities are disseminated intravascular coagulation (DIC) and heparin-associated thrombocytopenia (HAT).

Intravenous vitamin K, blood culture, urine culture, and q 12 hr platelet counts and coagulation times (to be drawn via peripheral venipuncture) are ordered. Platelet transfusion is not indicated.

> The patient's condition remained stable, and laboratory results did not change. She was extubated on postoperative day 2. The blood cultures were negative, but the urine culture grew $>10^5$ colonies of *Pseudomonas aeruginosa*. The patient then was given a third-generation cephalosporin.
>
> During early morning rounds on postoperative day 4, the medical student observed that the patient had mottled skin over the left calf. The left popliteal and dorsalis pedis pulses were thready. The patient was alert and complained of pain in the left leg. She had no dyspnea or chest or abdominal pain. Her temperature was 100° F, pulse was 96 and regular, and blood pressure was 100/78. On physical examination, the patient had no evidence of generalized or localized bleeding. Examination of the chest and heart was unremarkable in view of her postoperative condition. Abdominal examination revealed a normal liver and spleen and no bruit, tenderness, or mass. Femoral pulses were normal.
>
> - *The medical student asks your advice for management.*

The patient has had a sudden compromise of arterial blood flow on the fourth day after CPB. The diagnostic considerations are embolization and in situ arterial thrombosis. There is no evidence for abdominal aortic aneurysm or chronic atrial dysrhythmia, either of which could predispose the patient to arterial embolization. Serial cardiac enzymes have been followed, and there has been no acute myocardial infarction, which also might lead to embolization of thrombus from the left ventricle. Acute DIC, as a result of infection, surgical trauma, or occult myocardial infarction, also might be considered, but there is no overt evidence for any of these complications. PT, PTT, TT, and platelet count are ordered, with the following results:

Postoperative day 4: PT, PTT, TT normal
Platelet count 24,000/mm$^3$

Severe thrombocytopenia in the absence of abnormalities of the TT, PTT, and PT could be explained by several pathologic processes: HAT, drug-induced immune thrombocytopenia or bone marrow compromise, early acute DIC, and posttransfusion purpura. Although the patient has not been receiving therapeutic heparin postoperatively, the arterial line is heparinized. Furthermore, she had been heparinized during and after PTCA for 7 days. Now is the ideal time for onset of HAT.

You order immediate cessation of heparin in the arterial lines, discontinuation of the cephalosporin (can cause thrombocytopenia) and substitution of ampicillin, a platelet serotonin release assay, a CBC and peripheral blood smear (to look for evidence of microangiopathic changes of DIC), D-dimer level, blood cultures, and a hematology consultation.

A Doppler study of the leg confirmed the presence of a popliteal artery thrombus at the level of the midcalf. Infusion with urokinase was done to lyse the arterial thrombus. An echocardiogram showed no evidence for left ventricular thrombus. Evaluation of the peripheral blood smear was remarkable only for thrombocytopenia. The D-dimer level was mildly elevated, which you correctly interpreted as showing evidence for thrombosis, but not for DIC. The serotonin release assay was "strongly positive" for heparin antibodies. Blood cultures were again negative. During the next 12 hours, the patient's left leg warmed and pulses were easily palpated. The platelet count rose to 150,000/mm$^3$, and the patient became afebrile. The hematologist arrived for consultation that evening and found a recovering patient. She confirmed the diagnosis of HAT and commended you for your excellent management.

## CASE 2

A 40-year-old man with chronic diarrhea was hospitalized for massive ecchymoses of the abdominal wall and both thighs, associated with gastrointestinal bleeding. Except for broad-spectrum antibiotics, the patient had not had any medications. He had had no previous bleeding symptoms despite a number of hemostatic changes. Liver function test results were normal.

| *Laboratory Data* | *Patient* | *Normal* |
|---|---|---|
| Prothrombin time | 26 sec | 11-13.5 sec |
| PTT | 55 sec | 25-35 sec |
| Thrombin time | 15 sec | 13-18 sec |
| Bleeding time | 6 min | <9.5 min |
| Platelet count | 300,000/mm$^3$ | 150,000-450,000/mm$^3$ |
| Factor II | 20% | 70-130% |
| Factor V | 95% | 75-130% |
| Factor VII | 15% | 70-130% |
| Factor IX | 15% | 75-135% |
| Factor X | 25% | 70-130% |

- *What is the most likely cause of this patient's hemostatic abnormality? Discuss the clinical conditions responsible for this patient's bleeding disorder. What treatment modalities are available to correct this patient's hemostatic defect?*

This patient has acquired vitamin-K deficiency. Normally the liver synthesizes precursor protein Factors II, VII, IX, and X as well as protein C and protein S. These proteins require a postribosomal translational event that involves the gamma-carboxylation of the amino terminal glutamic acid of these proteins. Gamma-carboxylations of the glutamic acid residues confer normal binding of calcium ions to phospholipid surfaces (e.g., platelets), thus allowing for normal proteolytic activity. In the absence of gamma-carboxylation of glutamic acid, these proteins bind poorly with calcium with consequent reduced proteolytic activity. The enzyme involved is called gamma-glutamyl-carboxylase, and vitamin K functions as its coenzyme. The patient has a normal factor V level (which is synthesized in the liver but is not a vitamin K–dependent factor), signifying that liver disease is not the cause of the patient's coagulopathy. He has reduced endogenous sources of vitamin K, a consequence of chronic diarrhea and probable malabsorption, as well as eradication of the intestinal bacteria by antibiotics. A healthy diet, including leafy green vegetables, is necessary to maintain adequate levels of vitamin K. This patient should be treated with vitamin $K_1$ and fresh frozen plasma. As little as 1 mg of parenteral vitamin $K_1$ will correct the defect within 4 to 40 hours. The patient also should be evaluated for the cause of the chronic diarrhea and malabsorption syndrome.

**BIBLIOGRAPHY**

Bick RL. Hemostasis defects associated with cardiac surgery, prosthetic devices and other extracorporeal circuits. Semin Thromb Hemost 11:249, 1985.

Ferraris VA, Swanson E. Aspirin usage and perioperative blood loss in patients undergoing unexpected operations. Surg Gynecol Obstet 156:439, 1983.

Fuster V, Badimon L, Basfimon J, et al. Drugs interfering with platelet functions: Mechanisms and clinical relevance. In Verstraete M, Vermylen J, Lijnen HR, et al., eds. Thrombosis and Haemostasis (XIth Congress). 1987, p 349.

Hirsh J. Oral anticoagulant drugs. N Engl J Med 324:1865, 1991.

Kobrinsky NL, Israels ED, Gerrard JM, et al. Shortening of bleeding time by 1-deamino-8-D-arginine vasopressin in various bleeding disorders. Lancet 1:1145, 1984.

Manucci PM, Remuzzi G, Pusineri F, et al. Deamino-8-D-arginine vasopressin shortens the bleeding time in uremia. N Engl J Med 308:8, 1983.

Rapaport SI. Preoperative hemostatic evaluation: Which tests, if any? Blood 61:229, 1983.

Rizza CR. The treatment of hereditary and acquired bleeding disorders. In Walter Bowie EJ, Sharp AA, eds. Hemostasis and Thrombosis. London: Butterworth, 1985, p 259.

Salzman EW, Davies GC. Prophylaxis of venous thromboembolism: Analysis of cost/effectiveness. Ann Surg 191:201, 1980.

Triplett DA. Quantitative or functional disorders of platelets. In Triplett DA, ed. Platelet Function. Chicago: American Society of Clinical Pathology, 1978.

Vane JR, Anggard EE, Botting RM. Regulatory functions of the vascular endothelium. N Engl J Med 323:27, 1990.

# CHAPTER 35

## *Fluids and Electrolytes*

Roderick A. Barke

### CASE 1

A 72-year-old man was admitted to the emergency department from home with a 7-day history of increasing confusion, obtundation, and stupor 6 weeks after a distal ileal resection with primary anastomosis for a carcinoid tumor. The patient had no evidence of metastatic disease or carcinoid syndrome. He had a history of ethanol abuse and congestive heart failure with atrial fibrillation. Current medications included oral furosemide 40 mg daily and oral digoxin 0.25 mg daily. The patient's wife related a recent history of the patient having "the flu" 12 days prior to admission; symptoms consisted of anorexia, nausea, and vomiting. The family noted that although this brief illness had resolved, the patient had not been eating and drinking well. His medical history revealed admission 1 year earlier for left ventricular failure and pulmonary edema, demonstrated to be secondary to anterolateral myocardial infarction. The patient's recovery from that event was uncomplicated. On physical examination, the following pertinent information was noted:

Blood pressure: 90/60 mm Hg
Pulse: 118 beats/min; irregular, irregular
Respiratory rate: 10/min
Weight: 68 kg
HEENT: Dry mucous membranes
Skin: Poor skin turgor
Cardiovascular: No evidence of $S_3$ gallop; otherwise noncontributory
Respiratory: Rales bilaterally at bases
CNS: Stuporous white male with no focal findings

Laboratory examination revealed the following data:

Sodium: 165 mEq/L
Potassium: 3.5 mEq/L
BUN: 82 mg/100 ml
Creatinine: 2.3 mg/100 ml
Glucose: 165 mg/100 ml
Serum osmolality: 387 mOsm/kg
Serum lactate: 3.6 mmol/L
WBC: 8000/$mm^3$
Hg: 17 g/100 ml
ECG: Atrial fibrillation, poor R-wave progression in V1-V4, t-wave inversion in lateral precordial leads

This chapter can be studied in conjunction with *Essentials of Surgical Critical Care,* edited by Jerome H. Abrams and Frank B. Cerra (St. Louis: Quality Medical Publishing, Inc., 1993), Chapter 46.

This patient presents with a history and physical examination consistent with hyperosmolality with an unclear etiology. Presenting signs are tachycardia and hypotension. The working diagnosis would be hyperosmolality related to hypotonic fluid losses possibly associated with the use of loop diuretics and poor oral fluid intake. The patient is transferred to the SICU. The initial impression was that the osmolality may be excessively elevated compared to the electrolyte data. Accordingly, an osmolar gap was calculated with the following formula:

$$\text{Calculated serum osmolality} = 2(Na_s) + K_s + BUN/2.8 + Glucose/18$$

The calculated osmolality was 372 mOsm/kg compared with a measured osmolality of 387 mOsm/kg. These two figures agree closely enough to make the hypothesis of an unmeasured molecule contributing to the osmolality (i.e., ethanol) unlikely. The normal WBC suggests that an acute infectious complication following the brief viral illness is unlikely but cannot be excluded in an elderly patient. The initial approach to this patient should be to focus on the hypotension and tachycardia. Correction of the hyperosmolar hypernatremic condition is secondary in importance. Although it is assumed that the hypertension and tachycardia are the consequence of dehydration, other causes of hypotension should be considered. In this patient, fluid resuscitation should be initiated with 0.9% normal saline until a mean arterial pressure of >65 mm Hg and a urine output of >40 ml/hr has been achieved. With the history of previous congestive heart failure and myocardial infarction, it is likely that fluid resuscitation will be safer with central monitoring consisting of a Swan-Ganz catheter. On insertion of the Swan-Ganz catheter, the following data are obtained:

Pulse: 123
MAP: 55 mm Hg
Blood pressure: 88/40 mm Hg
Urine output: 15 ml/hr
CO/CI: 3.7 $L \cdot min^{-1}$/2.2 $L \cdot min^{-1} \cdot m^{-2}$
PA: 24/10 mm Hg
PCWP: 7 mm Hg
SVR: 2100 $dyne \cdot sec \cdot cm^{-5}$

The patient was given 1 L of 0.9% normal saline over 1 hour under constant observation of pulmonary artery (PA) and pulmonary capillary wedge (PCWP) pressures. At the end of this time, the PCWP remained <12 mm Hg and the mean arterial pressure (MAP) was 65 mm Hg. The decision was made to give another liter of 0.9% normal saline over 1 hour, and the following data were obtained:

Pulse: 95
MAP: 75 mm Hg
Blood pressure: 110/60 mm Hg
Urine output: 20 ml/hr
CO/CI: 4.2 $L \cdot min^{-1}$/2.5 $L \cdot min^{-1} \cdot m^{-2}$
PA: 31/14 mm Hg
PCWP: 12 mm Hg
SVR: 1400 $dyne \cdot sec \cdot cm^{-5}$

It is decided that the serum electrolyte data and osmolality should be repeated at this point to guide correction of the hyperosmolar state. The following data are obtained:

Sodium: 162 mEq/L
Potassium: 3.4 mEq/L
BUN: 78 mg/100 ml
Creatinine: 2.3 mg/100 ml
Glucose: 160 mg/100 ml
Serum osmolality: 363 mOsm/kg

The water deficit is calculated with the following formula:

$$\text{Water deficit (L)} = \{0.6\,[\text{BW(kg)}]\} \times \{[\text{plasma Na}^+\ (\text{mEq/L})]/[140\ (\text{mEq/L})] - 1\}$$

$$\text{Water deficit (L)} = \{0.6\,[68\ \text{kg}]\} \times \{[162\ \text{mEq/L}]/[140\ (\text{mEq/L})] - 1\}$$

The calculated water deficit is 6.4 L. It is of utmost importance, at this point in the patient's care, that several points be observed. First, since the patient presumably became hyperosmolar over several days, one should take at least 48 hours to rehydrate the patient and correct the hypernatremia to avoid the complications of rapid rehydration. Accordingly, 1.6 L of $D_5W$ over 12 hours is initiated in addition to a maintenance IV infusion. Secondly, the calculated fluid deficit should be taken as a rough approximation of the real deficit. Thus recalculation of the fluid requirements should be made every 12 hours to avoid complications.

## CASE 2

A 62-year-old man was admitted to the hospital with symptoms of sudden onset of left lower extremity pain and weakness. The symptoms began approximately 7 hours prior to admission. The patient had a history of recent onset of atrial fibrillation that was treated with digoxin and successfully converted to a sinus rhythm. The patient was otherwise in good health. On physical examination, the following pertinent findings were noted:

Blood pressure: 150/90 mm Hg
Pulse: 115 beats/min; regular
Respiratory rate: 13/min
Weight: 68 kg
Cardiovascular: Systolic ejection murmur consistent with aortic stenosis
Respiratory: Unremarkable
Extremities: Left lower extremity was noted to be cold and pale; an almost complete loss of sensation was noted below the knee

| *Pulses* | *RLL* | *LLE* |
|---|---|---|
| Femoral | 2+ | 0 |
| Popliteal | 1+ | 0 |
| Dorsalis pedis | 1+ | 0 |
| Posterior tibial | 0 | 0 |

Laboratory examination revealed the following pertinent findings:

Sodium: 142 mEq/L
Potassium: 4.8 mEq/L
BUN: 28 mg/100 ml
Creatinine: 1.2 mg/100 ml
Glucose: 130 mg/100 ml
WBC: 12,000/$mm^3$
Hg: 14 g/100 ml
ECG: Normal sinus rhythm, Q-waves in leads II, III, aVF

The diagnosis of acute left lower extremity arterial occlusion was made. The patient had angiography of the lower extremities, which confirmed the diagnosis of a common femoral occlusion. He was taken to the operating room, where a left femoral embolectomy was performed and arterial flow was reestablished. The patient was anticoagulated with heparin, and following his transfer to the postanesthesia recovery room, tall, peaked t-waves were noted on the rhythm strips. The electrolytes and ECG were repeated:

Sodium: 138 mEq/L
Potassium: 6.4 mEg/L
BUN: 22 mg/100 ml
Creatinine: 2.1 mg/100 ml
ECG: Tall, peaked t-waves, increased P-R interval
ABG: pH, 7.35; $P_{CO_2}$, 35 mm Hg; $P_{O_2}$, 154 mm Hg; $F_{IO_2}$, 40 mm Hg

The diagnosis of hyperkalemia was correctly obtained by a high index of suspicion and the presence of ECG abnormalities on the rhythm strips consistent with hyperkalemia. Almost simultaneously with the ECG evaluation, the patient is noted to have dark-brown urine. The presumptive diagnosis is myoglobinuria associated with left lower extremity compartment syndrome. Urinalysis is positive for hemoglobin but negative for RBCs, a finding consistent with myoglobinuria. Treatment of the hyperkalemia and myoglobinuria should begin immediately, while the patient is being prepared to return to the operating room for fasciotomy of the left lower extremity. Treatment for hyperkalemia usually includes the use of calcium gluconate to antagonize the membrane effects of increased potassium. However, in patients who are receiving digoxin treatment, calcium gluconate may precipitate malignant dysrhythmias. Thus in this patient, treatment of hyperkalemia is begun with 50 mEq of $NaHCO_3$ IV to redistribute the potassium into the intracellular space. An IV infusion is started with 100 mEq/L of $NaHCO_3$ at 100 ml/hr. Since the probability of acute renal failure is high at this point, volume must be administered carefully and monitored closely. In this particular patient, treatment with $NaHCO_3$ serves a dual purpose since alkalization of the urine (maintain urine pH $>7$) is also initial therapy for myoglobinuria. The patient is also given 12.5 to 25 g of mannitol IV and furosemide 80 mg IV to begin a brisk diuresis in an effort to prevent myoglobin-induced acute renal failure. Furosemide treatment again serves a dual purpose for both hyperkalemia and myoglobinuria. A glucose/insulin infusion is prepared consisting of 1 amp $D_{50}W$ and 10 units of regular insulin to be infused intravenously over 5 minutes. The rationale again is to redistribute the potassium into the cells. The patient is then taken to the operating room, where a four-compartment fasciotomy is performed on the left lower extremity.

# CHAPTER 36

# *Infection in the Immunocompromised Patient*

David L. Dunn

## CASE 1

A 26-year-old woman underwent cadaveric renal transplantation after developing chronic renal failure associated with chronic glomerulonephritis. Routine immunosuppression, consisting of cyclosporine, azathioprine, prednisone, and an initial 7-day course of antilymphocyte globulin, was implemented and the patient's serum creatinine concentration decreased to 1.4. Two months after successful renal transplantation, the patient's serum creatinine concentration rose to 2.8 and a percutaneous renal allograft biopsy demonstrated acute tubular interstitial and mild vascular rejection. An initial increase in oral steroids failed to reverse the rejection process, and murine monoclonal antibody OKT3 therapy was instituted for 10 days, and a gradual reduction in the oral steroid dosage was implemented. The initial steroid dose was 2 mg/kg/day, and this amount was reduced by .25 mg/kg/day every 3 days. The patient's creatinine concentration decreased to 1.6, and she was discharged 1 day after receiving her last dose of OKT3. Two days after discharge, the patient developed a low-grade fever (100.8° F orally), nausea, and vomiting. She was initially seen at an emergency department near her home and was diagnosed as having a "viral syndrome." The nausea persisted, the patient developed intermittent vomiting, and then presented for further evaluation.

On physical examination, the patient was found to be in no acute distress and was noted as having minimal (if any) abdominal tenderness. Laboratory studies revealed a hemoglobin of 11,400/mm$^3$, a WBC count of 28,500 cells/mm$^3$, and a normal differential. The serum creatinine concentration was 1.9, and the serum amylase and bilirubin were normal. A CXR film and flat plate and upright radiographic study of the abdomen were obtained, both of which revealed a crescent-shaped radiolucent area beneath the left hemidiaphragm, which the radiologist thought could be consistent with pneumoperitoneum. The radiologist recommended obtaining a Gastrogafin or barium upper GI series, a Gastrogafin or barium enema, or both.

- *What further diagnostic and treatment measures would you institute at this time?*

Delay of diagnosis of an intra-abdominal catastrophe in an immunosuppressed patient is associated with a marked increase in mortality. It is extremely likely that this patient has developed a perforated viscus, and three different forms of therapy are necessary to treat this problem: (1) expeditious fluid resuscitation and hemodynamic monitoring, (2) empiric antimicrobial

This chapter can be studied in conjunction with *Essentials of Surgical Critical Care,* edited by Jerome H. Abrams and Frank B. Cerra (St. Louis: Quality Medical Publishing, Inc., 1993), Chapters 2, 27, 40, *47,* and 48. Italicized number indicates the main chapter reference.

agent therapy, and (3) exploratory laparotomy in order to establish "source control." In this situation it is rarely necessary (and may be hazardous) to pursue further diagnostic studies. Exploratory laparotomy almost invariably will reveal the source of perforation. Although it is by no means clear that a transplanted kidney is more sensitive to hemodynamic changes than the normal native kidneys, every effort must be made to protect the transplanted allograft. Assessment of adequacy of fluid hydration should be established by placement of a urinary catheter and a central venous line. If any question exists regarding the adequacy of central venous pressure monitoring, a Swan-Ganz catheter should be inserted. Administration of a diuretic and mannitol also may be of benefit.

In this situation empiric antimicrobial agent therapy is based on treatment for what might be termed the "worst case scenario." In a patient who suffers perforation of a hollow viscus, the worst case would be perforation of the distal colon because: (1) a large number of microorganisms are present, and (2) a large proportion of anaerobic-to-aerobic bacteria act together to cause synergistic infections. For that reason empiric antibacterial therapy should be directed against both aerobes and anaerobes. The "gold standard" therapy in this situation consists of either clindamycin or metronidazole (antianaerobic therapy) plus an aminoglycoside. Over the last several years, however, the use of selected second- and third-generation cephalosporins, extended-spectrum penicillins plus a beta-lactamase inhibitor, and carbapenems as single agents have provided equivalent results. Single agents must be selected carefully to ensure that they possess both an antianaerobic and an antiaerobic spectrum of activity. Many of these agents are attractive in this situation because of their lack of nephrotoxicity. A plethora of combinations of agents also exists. For instance, use of clindamycin plus a monobactam or an antianaerobic agent combined with either an extended-spectrum penicillin or a third-generation cephalosporin that lacks antianaerobic coverage but possesses excellent antiaerobic coverage also would be suitable.

The patient received a carbapenem agent intravenously after having adequate fluid resuscitation. Excellent urine output was obtained, and the patient underwent exploratory laparotomy. Exploration revealed a modicum of purulent material and a perforation of the midsigmoid colon with minimal inflammation. Cultures for aerobes, anaerobes, and fungi were obtained at this time, and a Gram's stain also was requested. Following sigmoid resection, colostomy, and Hartmann's procedure, the abdomen was then copiously lavaged initially with fluid containing a first-generation cephalosporin and subsequently containing amphotericin B. The wound was left open to heal by secondary intention or delayed primary closure.

This patient probably should receive a minimum of 7 to 10 days' administration of the intravenous antimicrobial agent. Studies in normal individuals indicate that shorter courses are feasible, but this hypothesis has not been tested in immunosuppressed patients. In addition, the life-threatening nature of this disease process mandates a decrease in immunosuppressive therapy. In general, it is prudent to withhold either cyclosporine or azathioprine and maintain the patient on a maintenance dose of prednisone (generally 0.15 to 0.25 mg/kg/day).

The culture results revealed heavy growth of *Escherichia coli* and *Klebsiella pneumoniae* (both sensitive to the carbapenem agent) and *Bacteroides distasonis* (anaerobic sensitivities were not performed), *Streptococcus faecalis,* and a moderate growth of *Candida albicans.* This patient had regained near-normal bowel function, was afebrile, and was feeling well.

- *How would you adjust the patient's antimicrobial agent regimen?*

This patient is doing exceedingly well. On that basis alone, radical adjustments in the antimicrobial agent regimen, in general, are not justifiable. Since carbapenem agents do not cover

*Streptococcus faecalis,* if this patient exhibited evidence of ongoing infection, it would be prudent to add either ampicillin or vancomycin to the regimen. The presence of *Candida albicans,* however, within the peritoneal fluid is of concern even in the patient who is exhibiting recovery. In immunosuppressed patients, the presence of this pathogen in peritoneal fluid culture is associated with a high mortality unless it is treated with amphotericin B. Therefore this patient should receive a minimum of 350 to 500 mg of amphotericin B intravenously. Other antifungal agents (e.g., triazole, fluconazole) may be efficacious in this setting, but this hypothesis has yet to be proven. Serious fungal infections such as *Candida* peritonitis should continue to be treated with amphotericin B. Renal toxicity generally can be avoided with conservative daily dosing and every-other-day dosing regimens. The fact that this patient may be receiving cyclosporine, vancomycin, and amphotericin B simultaneously should lead the clinician to anticipate potential problems with drug-related nephrotoxicity. With that in mind, it would be prudent to discontinue cyclosporine and continue to administer azathioprine and perhaps select ampicillin in place of vancomycin, if a decision should be made to implement antienterococcal therapy.

## CASE 2

A 33-year-old gentleman who developed type I diabetes mellitus at the age of 16, and who also developed renal failure, progressive retinopathy, and neuropathy, underwent combined cadaveric renal and pancreatic transplantation. The pancreatic allograft contained a segment of duodenum that was anastomosed to the bladder for the purpose of monitoring pancreatic exocrine drainage and urinary amylase. The patient developed concordant renal and pancreatic allograft rejection on three occasions within a period of 5½ months; each time the treatment was an antilymphocyte antibody (either ALG or OKT3) administered for 10 to 14 days. Serologic studies of the donor and the recipient revealed the presence of antibodies to cytomegalovirus (CMV) in the donor but not in the patient. Three weeks after the last successful course of antirejection therapy, the patient developed persistent fever to 102.6° F orally, rigors, severe myalgias, and lethargy. The patient was admitted for a diagnostic evaluation. The patient had been receiving prophylactic trimethoprim-sulfamethoxazole and acyclovir.

In an immunosuppressed transplant patient, the degree of global immunosuppression is associated with an increased frequency of bacterial, fungal, and viral infections. At this juncture, this patient requires an extensive diagnostic evaluation and most likely will require fluid resuscitation and hemodynamic support. The fact that this patient is somewhat dyspneic should lead one to focus on the pulmonary system after (1) obtaining an adequate history, (2) performing a physical examination, and (3) ordering routine laboratory studies, including specimens of blood and urine for performance of Gram's stain and aerobic, anaerobic, and acid-fast bacterial, fungal, and viral cultures. CMV-enhanced shell vial analysis (rapid antigen) can be performed upon blood and sputum. A sputum sample also should be sent for Gram's, potassium hydroxide, and Ziehl-Neelsen stains, and cultures for aerobic and acid-fast bacilli, fungi, and viruses should be done. Arterial blood gases should be obtained in conjunction with a CXR examination.

The arterial blood gases revealed mild acidosis and hypoxemia, and the CXR film showed bilaterally hazy, diffuse infiltrates.

- *How would you proceed with the diagnostic evaluation of this patient?*

The evaluation for pulmonary infection in this patient should be pursued aggressively. Bronchoscopy with bronchoalveolar lavage should be performed, and the samples obtained should be sent for Gram's, methenamine silver, and Giemsa stains, and aerobic and acid-fast bacterial, fungal, and viral cultures should be done. In addition, the CMV-enhanced shell vial analysis should be performed. If necessary, the patient should undergo endotracheal intubation and ventilatory support if the degree of hypoxemia is such that the bronchoscopic procedure would be hazardous. It may be possible to avoid performance of bronchoalveolar lavage in selected cases, however, if several extrapulmonary sources reveal the presence of a specific pathogen that appears to be disseminated or if analysis of the sputum samples reveals clear results.

> The patient underwent bronchoscopy and bronchoalveolar lavage. No endobronchial lesions were noted; nor was purulent material present. Occasional Gram-positive cocci in chains were noted on the Gram's stain, and the potassium hydroxide preparation revealed hyphal forms with septations. The CMV-enhanced shell vial assay was positive at 18 hours. The patient had required intubation and mechanical ventilation for respiratory support.
>
> - *What therapy would you institute?*

This patient has concurrent life-threatening fungal and viral infections. Even prior to absolute confirmation via cultural data, empiric antifungal and antiviral therapy is warranted. This patient most likely has developed these infections as a consequence of repeated courses of antirejection therapy. At this point, it is necessary to attempt to save the patient's life, even at the risk of incurring rejection and loss of both the renal and pancreatic allografts. If these results should occur, this patient can survive on hemodialysis and exogenous insulin. Three forms of therapy are indicated: (1) IV amphotericin B, (2) IV ganciclovir, and (3) a reduction in immunosuppression. I generally favor the addition of 5-fluorocytocine and rifampin to amphotericin B for treatment of *Aspergillus* infection. Obtaining antifungal agent sensitivities of the organism also may be helpful. If amphotericin B resistance should be present, therapy with itraconazole could be considered. Amphotericin B, however, remains the mainstay of therapy for all patients with serious, life-threatening fungal infections. Ganciclovir therapy should be instituted at a dose of 5 mg/kg every 12 hours in patients with normal renal function. CMV hyperimmune globulin and normal globulin preparations that contain antibody activity directed against CMV may be of benefit, although this effect remains unproven. This patient may not survive without a concurrent substantial reduction immunosuppressive therapy. With life-threatening infection, discontinuing cyclosporine and azathioprine and administering only maintenance doses of prednisone (7.5 to 10 mg/day in adults) is warranted. Finally, prolonged antifungal therapy will be required in this patient. This therapy most likely will consist of 1 to 1.5 g of amphotericin B as the total dose. Incidentally, this patient most likely has developed the diffuse bronchoalveolar form of *Aspergillus* infection and will not require any type of surgical extirpation because no discrete focus is present. If a discrete mass should develop, initial antifungal therapy followed by surgical extirpation should be considered.

# PART FIVE

# *COMMON SICU PROCEDURES*

# CHAPTER 37

# *Bronchoscopy*

**Marshall I. Hertz • Paul Gustafson**

## CASE 1

The patient was a 45-year-old man who was the driver of an automobile involved in a head-on collision. He required extensive operative management of multiple injuries, including a lacerated liver and a fractured femur. The estimated blood loss was 2400 ml, and he received 2000 ml of crystalloid solution, six units of packed RBCs, and four units of fresh frozen plasma. The patient was brought to the SICU. He remained intubated and mechanically ventilated but had improving arterial oxygenation over the first 24 postoperative hours. However, on postoperative day 2, deteriorating oxygenation was noted with an increase in $F_{IO_2}$ requirement from 0.3 to 0.7. A CXR film demonstrated diffuse bilateral pulmonary infiltrates. A diagnosis of adult respiratory distress syndrome (ARDS) was made, and positive end-expiratory pressure was begun. A Swan-Ganz catheter was placed. The pulmonary artery pressure was 34/18 mm Hg, the pulmonary capillary wedge pressure was 13 mm Hg, and the right atrial pressure was 8 mm Hg. The cardiac output was 7.3 L/min, and the calculated systemic vascular resistance was 930 dyne · sec · $cm^{-5}$. The patient remained stable until postoperative day 14, when fever and a decrease in blood pressure to 90/60 mm Hg were noted. The cardiac output was then 12.4 L/min, and the systemic vascular resistance was 450 dyne · sec · $cm^{-5}$. The CXR film demonstrated a new right lower lobe infiltrate. Bronchoscopy and bronchoalveolar lavage were performed. The bronchoscopist observed no sputum in the airways. The bronchoalveolar lavage fluid was cloudy, and the WBC differential showed 64% neutrophils (normal <10% neutrophils). Gram-negative rods were seen on the Gram's stain, and cultures of BAL fluid grew *Klebsiella pneumoniae*. Therapy with ticarcillin and tobramycin was begun, and over the ensuing 72 hours the fever resolved, with improvement in the blood pressure and increased systemic vascular resistance to 850 dyne · sec · $cm^{-5}$.

This patient developed a nosocomial Gram-negative pneumonia as a complication of ARDS and prolonged intubation. Gram-negative pneumonias are common in this setting and need not be associated with increased sputum production. In this case the pneumonia was associated with systemic inflammatory response syndrome (SIRS), consisting of fever, decreased systemic vascular resistance, and increased cardiac output. SIRS frequently occurs in patients with ARDS and may or may not be associated with an infection. When infection is present, a pulmonary source is common. In ARDS patients in whom sepsis syndrome begins or intensifies, our practice

This chapter can be studied in conjunction with *Essentials of Surgical Critical Care,* edited by Jerome H. Abrams and Frank B. Cerra (St. Louis: Quality Medical Publishing, Inc., 1993), Chapters 1, 2, 5, 25, 27, and *48*. Italicized number indicates the main chapter reference.

is to perform BAL (if the patient's condition permits) to identify nosocomially acquired or reactivated endogenous (i.e., herpes simplex virus) infectious organisms.

## CASE 2

A 75-year-old man underwent an uncomplicated carotid endarterectomy for transient ischemic episodes associated with a carotid bruit. The patient was extubated in the recovery room and transferred to a general surgical unit. He did well with the exception of nocturnal confusion until postoperative day 3, when he developed a cough without sputum production or fever. A CXR film demonstrated volume loss of the left lower lobe. Pulmonary consultation was obtained, and percussion with postural drainage and incentive spirometry were recommended. The following day the patient experience the acute onset of dyspnea. Breath sounds over the left hemithorax were decreased. The arterial $Po_2$ was 40 mm Hg, the $Pco_2$ was 33 mm Hg, and the pH was 7.46.

The patient was transferred to the SICU, and endotracheal intubation was performed. Repeat CXR film showed complete atelectasis of the left lung (Fig. 37-1). Flexible fiberoptic bronchoscopy (FFB) demonstrated mucus completely obstructing the left main bronchus. Following removal of the mucus by suction through the FFB, a CXR film showed prompt reexpansion of the left lung (Fig. 37-2). The patient was extubated the following day and had an uncomplicated hospital course.

This case illustrates the common postoperative problem of atelectasis, which may range in severity from trivial to catastrophic. Measures to prevent atelectasis include postoperative incentive spirometry, cough and deep breathing, and early ambulation. Especially in patients who are not producing sputum, it is often unclear whether atelectasis is caused by mucus obstruction of central airways or whether it is functional in nature. Therefore percussion and postural drainage generally are instituted for 24 hours and then discontinued if sputum production does

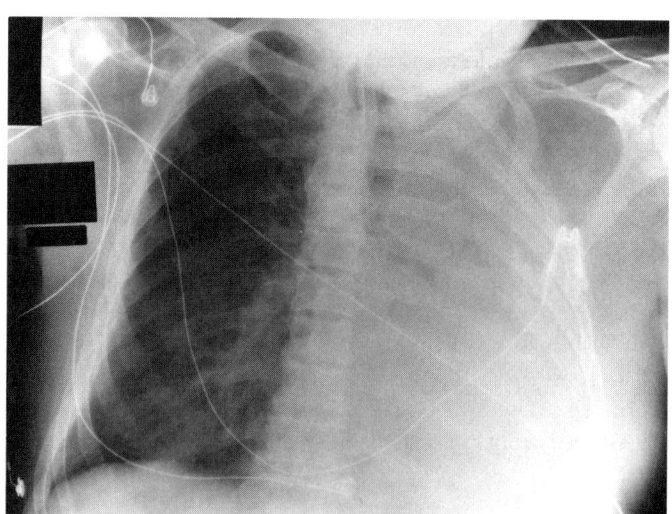

FIG 37-1

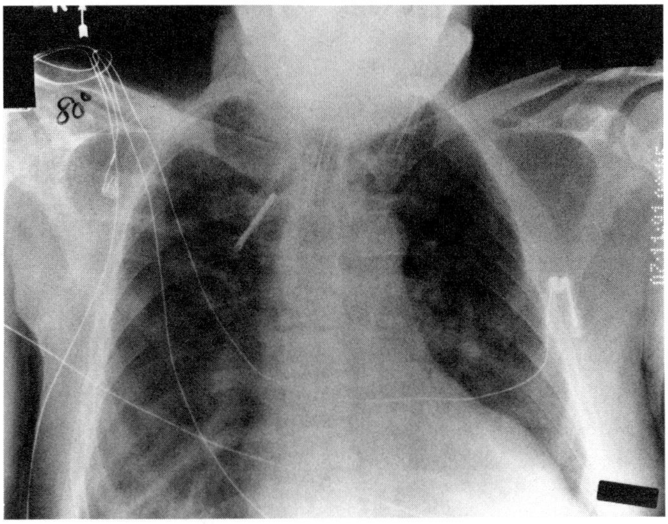

FIG 37-2

not increase. In most cases conservative measures will be sufficient to prevent major atelectasis of a lobe or a lung. For cases in which lobar atelectasis occurs or in which respiratory deterioration is associated with atelectasis, particularly when breath sounds to the atelectatic area are absent, FFB can be of therapeutic use.

■ ■ ■

FFB is an important diagnostic and therapeutic tool. Common uses of FFB in the critical care setting include evaluation and treatment of hemoptysis, treatment of atelectasis caused by mucus plugging, and obtaining specimens of lower respiratory tract secretions from patients with suspected pneumonia. Of the many procedures that can be accomplished transbronchoscopically, bronchoalveolar lavage is the most useful technique for the diagnosis of suspected lower respiratory tract infection because of its safety and diagnostic accuracy. A thorough prebronchoscopy evaluation is necessary to identify contraindications. The contraindications include factors mandating endotracheal intubation before the procedure and factors that contraindicate FFB even in intubated patients, such as hemodynamic instability and severe hypoxemia. Common complications of FFB include widening of the arterial-to-alveolar oxygen gradient and bronchospasm. Complications of bronchoalveolar lavage include hypoxemia, fever, and pneumonia.

# CHAPTER 38

## *Care of Central Lines*

Steven D. Eyer

### CASE

A 47-year-old alcoholic man was admitted to the SICU with a 2-day history of severe abdominal pain. The patient was severely dehydrated and demonstrated a rigid, exquisitely tender abdomen. Upright CXR film revealed free intraperitoneal air. Perforated duodenal ulcer with generalized peritonitis was suspected. A triple-lumen catheter was placed under emergency conditions, using sterile protocol in the left subclavian vein. Follow-up CXR examination revealed no complications of central venous catheter placement and good position of the catheter tip at the junction of the right atrium and superior vena cava. Central venous pressure was zero. Vigorous hydration and preoperative broad-spectrum antibiotics were given. At laparotomy, perforated duodenal ulcer with generalized peritonitis was found. Cultures were obtained. Vagotomy and pyloroplasty with copious peritoneal irrigation were performed. The patient was stable throughout the procedure and on completion was returned to the SICU.

On arrival, the patient was alert, responsive, and intubated. Vital signs were: pulse, 100; blood pressure, 120/70; central venous pressure, 6 mm Hg, and temperature 102° F. The patient was breathing with the ventilator at a rate of 12. Urine output was 100 ml/hr. Blood gases were normal, and serum lactate concentration was 1.5 mmol.

- *Would you change the patient's central line?*

The central line should not be changed for the increased body temperature or because it was placed on an emergency basis preoperatively. Despite being placed as an emergency, it was done with aseptic protocol. If hyperalimentation is begun, a new central venous catheter should be exchanged by guidewire technique because a port was not "saved for TPN" when the triple-lumen catheter was placed. Exchange of the central line before beginning hyperalimentation will reduce the risk of complications.

The patient did well postoperatively. He was extubated on postoperative day 1 and transferred to the ward on postoperative day 2 with resolution of his fever. Peritoneal cultures were positive for multiple Gram-negative aerobic bacilli. Hyperalimentation with enriched branch-chain formula and antibiotics was begun on postoperative day 2. Abdominal discomfort improved daily. On postoperative day 5, the patient suddenly became confused and diaphoretic. He had a temperature of 102.5° F with thick yellow sputum on coughing. Right-sided breath sounds were markedly diminished. His nasogastric tube appeared functional.

This chapter can be studied in conjunction with *Essentials of Surgical Critical Care*, edited by Jerome H. Abrams and Frank B. Cerra (St. Louis: Quality Medical Publishing, Inc., 1993), Chapter 49.

The patient's abdomen was benign, and his open wound was clean. There was no extremity swelling. An arterial blood gas and CXR film were obtained, and 100% oxygen was started by mask. Blood gases were: pH, 7.55; $P_{CO_2}$, 27 mm Hg; and $P_{O_2}$, 48 mm Hg. CXR film revealed decreased right thoracic volume with consolidation and air bronchograms in the right lower lobe. The patient was intubated and transferred to the SICU. Copious thick secretions were removed with suctioning and breath sounds improved in the right lower lung fields.

- *What plans do you have now? Should the central line be changed?*

The patient's symptoms and acute pulmonary infiltrate likely represent pneumonia. Aspiration is possible, but the nasogastric tube seems to be working well, and there was no evidence for gastric content on endotracheal suctioning. Cultures should be obtained, and adjustment of antibiotics should be considered. Postoperative pneumonia and atelectasis following upper abdominal surgery is, unfortunately, common. The patient has an obvious source of infection, and the central line should not be changed. However, the possibility of line infection is not entirely excluded. If the fever persists despite resolution of the pneumonia, the line should be cultured. If the percutaneous puncture site appears clear, the central venous catheter may be exchanged over a guidewire.

PART SIX

# *MEASUREMENT AND INTERPRETATION OF DATA*

# CHAPTER 39

# *Blood Pressure Monitoring*

Jerome H. Abrams

## CASE

A 64-year-old man was admitted to the SICU following repair of an abdominal aortic aneurysm. The postoperative orders included infusion of sodium nitroprusside to keep the systolic blood pressure between 100 and 140 mm Hg. You were informed that the arterial blood pressure line and the blood pressure obtained by cuff do not agree. The arterial line read a systolic blood pressure of 165 mm Hg, and the cuff pressure was only 125 mm Hg. You were asked which blood pressure to use to guide sodium nitroprusside therapy.

The situation in which the arterial blood pressure obtained both by continuous blood pressure monitoring with an arterial catheter and by a blood pressure cuff do not agree is not uncommon. First verify that the blood pressure obtained by blood pressure cuff is equal in both arms. If the blood pressure is equal in both arms, you should check the damping characteristics of the arterial blood pressure line.

You performed a square-wave test by suddenly opening and occluding the continuous infusion device attached to the arterial line. The results are shown in Fig. 39-1.

- *What is your approach at this point?*

This chapter can be studied in conjunction with *Essentials of Surgical Critical Care,* edited by Jerome H. Abrams and Frank B. Cerra (St. Louis: Quality Medical Publishing, Inc., 1993), Chapter 52.

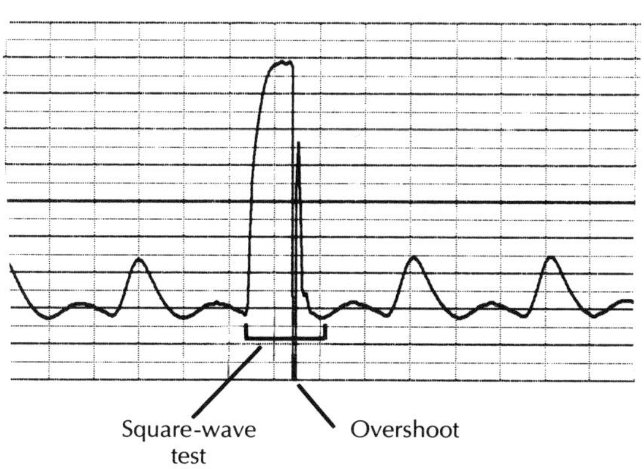


**FIG 39-1** Waveform of blood pressure when arterial line and cuff do not agree.

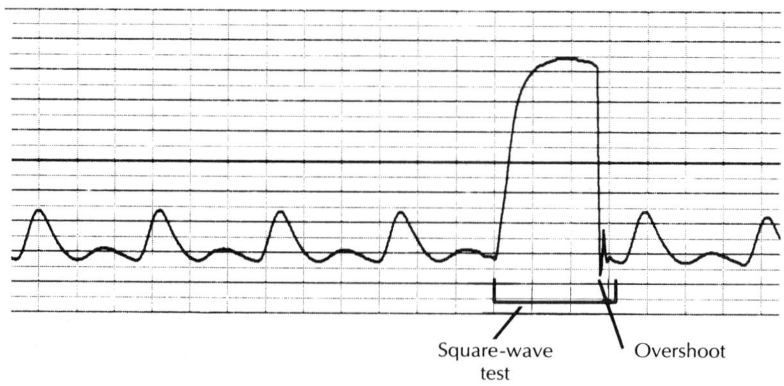


**FIG 39-2** Waveform of blood pressure after auxiliary damping is added.

The square-wave test shows suboptimal damping. The signal demonstrates both excessive overshoot and ringing. Both of these features are characteristic of an underdamped system. In your institution, an adjustable damping device is included with the arterial blood pressure monitoring device. You increase the damping until the square-wave test is improved.

> With additional damping, you obtained another square-wave test. The results are shown in Fig. 39-2.
>
> - *What is your approach at this point?*

The square-wave test, performed after auxiliary damping is added to the measurement system, shows an overshoot of <10% of the amplitude of the square-wave signal. In addition, the ringing is reduced. These characteristics are consistent with clinically optimal damping. When these characteristics are achieved, a reasonable compromise between amplitude response and time response for the system is reached.

> After adjustment of the arterial line, the systolic arterial blood pressure read 127 mm Hg. The blood pressure cuff remained at 125 mm Hg.

The most likely occurrence when the arterial line shows a higher value than the blood pressure cuff is that the arterial line is underdamped. Commonly used configurations for arterial blood pressure monitoring are frequently underdamped. The situation in which the blood pressure determined by arterial line is less than the cuff pressure is more complicated. Usually the damping of the arterial pressure monitoring system is excessive. Careful examination for the presence of air bubbles in the pressure line, sharp bends in the catheter tubing, or excessive additional damping should be performed.

# CHAPTER 40

# *Respiratory Monitoring*

Ian J. Gilmour

## CASE 1

A 48-year-old woman weighing 94 kg was on a general surgical ward 2 days after having had an abdominal hysterectomy and bilateral salpingo-oophorectomy with node dissection for uterine carcinoma. The initial procedure had been uneventful, but approximately 36 hours postoperatively the patient began to complain of increasing abdominal pain. Additional analgesia failed to relieve her discomfort. Physical and laboratory findings suggested a diagnosis of postoperative hemorrhage, which was confirmed at laparotomy. A tear in the right iliac vein was repaired, and the patient was returned to the SICU for further care. On admission, she was somnolent and controlled on mechanical ventilation with settings of: $V_T$, 900 ml; RR, 10; PEEP, 5 cm $H_2O$; and $FIO_2$, 0.5. Her temperature was 101° F. Arterial blood gases were: pH, 7.44; $PaCO_2$, 34; $PaO_2$, 106; other lab data were unremarkable. The patient was monitored with pulse oximetry and infrared capnometry with the plan of weaning her from positive pressure ventilation as she became more responsive. Approximately 5 hours after admission, the nurse heard the pressure alarm on the ventilator and observed that the patient seemed to be in respiratory distress.

- *What is your differential diagnosis?*

The patient is an obese female whose first surgical procedure was more than 2 days prior to her ICU admission. Consideration must be given to several possible diagnoses, weighted by available laboratory and clinical data. The differential diagnosis includes: pain/anxiety, primary pulmonary dysfunction such as bronchospasm, adult respiratory distress syndrome, atelectasis, fluid overload, pulmonary embolism, and pneumothorax.

Observation of the patient revealed that she was overdriving the ventilator to a respiratory rate of 20 to 25 breaths/min and that the pressure alarms resulted from asynchrony between patient effort and ventilator response. She was awake, diaphoretic, tachycardic, and obviously in severe respiratory distress. Apart from small areas of bronchial breath sounds over both lower lobes posteriorly, chest auscultation revealed no other diagnostic findings. Her $SpO_2$ was 91%, and $PetCO_2$ was 26 mm Hg.

- *Do these data narrow your differential diagnosis?*

---

This chapter can be studied in conjunction with *Essentials of Surgical Critical Care,* edited by Jerome H. Abrams and Frank B. Cerra (St. Louis: Quality Medical Publishing, Inc., 1993), Chapters 12, 22, 25, 26, 27, and *54*. Italicized number indicates the main chapter reference.

The observation that the ventilator pressure alarm was responding to asynchrony between patient and machine means that airway pressure changes could not be used as a specific diagnostic tool. Diaphoresis, tachycardia, tachypnea, and patient anxiety/distress are worrisome but too nonspecific to be helpful. Findings on auscultation make bronchospasm and significant fluid overload less probable. Given the uncertainty about airway pressure and the lack of reliability of auscultation as a diagnostic tool for this condition, pneumothorax is still a consideration. Particularly helpful are the patterns of change in pulse oximetry and capnometry. Your knowledge of the oxyhemoglobin dissociation curve tells you that the $Spo_2$ of 91 correlates with a $Pao_2$ in the low 60s. The nurse confirmed that $Spo_2$ had fallen significantly since admission. When the $Petco_2$ of 26 is compared with the initial blood gas, the $Paco_2$-$Petco_2$ gradient is 13. Pulmonary embolism is a real possibility, although it must be kept in mind that with her tachypnea, the patient might well have a true respiratory alkalosis and a "normal" $Paco_2$-$Petco_2$.

Stat arterial blood gases were drawn and orders written for immediate CXR examination and duplex ultrasonography of the lower extremities. Although the CXR film revealed only bilateral streaky lower lobe infiltrates, the arterial blood gas results were interesting: pH, 7.35; $Paco_2$, 45; and $Pao_2$, 62. The $Paco_2$-$Petco_2$ gradient was, in fact, 19; the low $Spo_2$ was confirmed. The most likely diagnosis, which would explain combined hypoxia and increased dead space, is pulmonary embolism (PE). Duplex ultrasound findings of impeded flow above the right femoral vein supported the diagnosis. A subsequent V/Q scan revealed several small, unmatched defects in the right, middle, and lower lobes. The combination of ultrasound data and V/Q scan findings made the diagnosis of pulmonary embolism likely, over 90%. Given this high probability, a pulmonary arteriogram was not considered necessary. The patient was treated appropriately and discharged from the hospital on postoperative day 15.

The divergence of $Paco_2$ and $Petco_2$ with increasing V/Q mismatch is exemplified in this case. These findings occur when alveolar dead space increases and expired gas comes from both perfused and underperfused alveoli. This clinical situation emphasizes the unreliability of $Petco_2$ as a substitute for $Paco_2$. Although an actual elevation of $Paco_2$ with pulmonary embolism is unusual, it may occur with massive PE and in those cases in which response to elevated carbon dioxide may be depressed, as in this case, following administration of narcotics for postoperative pain.

## CASE 2

The patient was a 62-year-old man weighing 60 kg who presented to the emergency department complaining of dyspnea and chest pain. The chest pain quickly subsided following administration of oxygen (4 L by nasal prongs) and sublingual nitroglycerin. Although his pain resolved, some dyspnea remained. CXR film revealed a patchy infiltrate, primarily involving the right lower lobe, and large lung volumes with somewhat flattened diaphragms. The patient stated that he had been unwell for several days. Further questioning uncovered a smoking history of 85 pack-years and a chronic productive cough. Although the patient had been told by his physician that he had "emphysema," he had continued to smoke. He was admitted to the SICU.

- *How would you monitor this patient's respiratory status?*

At this point, you suspect that the patient's underlying pathology is a combination of chronic bronchitis and atherosclerotic coronary artery disease. It is difficult to determine whether his current deterioration is primarily the result of an acute exacerbation of his chronic obstructive pulmonary disease or whether the primary problem is cardiac. Initial monitoring with pulse oximetry, cardiac monitor, and an arterial line would be appropriate, with consideration given to invasive cardiac monitoring with a Swan-Ganz catheter.

> Initial arterial blood gases were: pH, 7.34; $Pa_{CO_2}$, 56; $Pa_{O_2}$, 62 on 4 L nasal $O_2$. A nitroglycerin infusion was begun. Orders were written for bronchodilators by aerosol, deep breathing and coughing, and broad-spectrum antibiotics. The patient was febrile. In spite of these measures, his dyspnea increased and he began to use his accessory muscles of ventilation. $Sp_{O_2}$ dropped below 90%, and chest pain recurred. Arterial blood gases at this time were: pH, 7.25; $Pa_{CO_2}$, 72; $Pa_{O_2}$, 56. The physician caring for the patient intubated and mechanically ventilated him.
>
> - *What ventilatory measurements will be especially important to monitor at this point?*

Special consideration needs to be given to airway pressure monitoring along with $Pet_{CO_2}/Sp_{O_2}$ and frequent arterial blood gases. This patient will require continuous blood pressure measurement. Assessment of cardiac function and oxygen consumption also are indicated.

> The patient was intubated orally using succinyl dicholine and IV sedation with midazolam. Immediately following intubation, blood pressure dropped but responded to IV fluids. Initial ventilator settings were: tidal volume, 750; respiratory rate, 12; PEEP, 0; and $F_{IO_2}$, 0.6. Over the next 30 minutes, the respiratory rate gradually increased to 15 to 18 breaths/min, with frequent patient inspiratory efforts to which the ventilator did not respond. The machine rate was correspondingly increased to 18 breaths/min. The pressure alarm sounded frequently as $P_{max}$ exceeded 60 cm $H_2O$. The patient gradually became hypotensive and tachycardic. He continued to use his accessory muscles of expiration. He was diaphoretic and his extremities were cold and clammy. On auscultation, rhonchi were heard throughout expiration. The pulse oximeter alarmed frequently, and $Sp_{O_2}$ was 85% to 87%. $Pet_{CO_2}$ was approximately 35 mm Hg, and the alveolar plateau of the capnogram was irregular and quite steep. A Swan-Ganz catheter was placed. Pulmonary artery occlusion pressure (PAOP) was recorded as 28 mm Hg. Consideration was given to a diagnosis of tension pneumothorax. CXR examination and arterial blood gases were ordered.

Attempting to assess airway pressures under these circumstances is very difficult because it is almost impossible to obtain reliable baseline data during asynchrony of ventilator and patient. Almost certainly the cause of the patient's difficulty is excessive intrathoracic gas. The physician must determine whether this gas is intrapulmonary or interpleural. The observation that the patient deteriorated gradually as he awoke from sedation following intubation and his respiratory rate increased suggests that he might be better maintained on completely controlled mechanical ventilation using muscle relaxants* and sedation. Careful attention should be paid to intravascular volume and other components of his cardiac function.

> On initiation of paralysis and sedation, ventilator settings were: tidal volume, 750; respiratory rate, 18; $F_{IO_2}$, 1; PEEP, 0. $P_{max}$ was 58 cm $H_2O$; $P_{ei}$ was 47 cm $H_2O$. Rhonchi continued to be heard throughout expiration. The patient remained mildly hypotensive and tachycardic. PAOP was 20 mm Hg. The CXR film was unchanged; no pneumothorax was seen. Repeat blood gases were: pH, 7.28; $Pa_{CO_2}$, 68; $Pa_{O_2}$, 68; $Pet_{CO_2}$, 39. Intrinsic PEEP was assessed at end-expiration and determined to be 15 cm $H_2O$. The respiratory rate was lowered to 10 breaths/min. $P_{max}$ dropped to 40 cm $H_2O$, and $P_{ei}$ fell to 30 cm $H_2O$. Intrinsic PEEP at end-expiration was 8 cm $H_2O$ and PAOP was 12 mm Hg. At this point, resuscitation with intra-

---

**Editor's note:* Use of muscle relaxants should be given careful thought. Absence of spontaneous cough, muscle wasting, and prolonged paralysis following long-term infusion of certain agents present important risks.

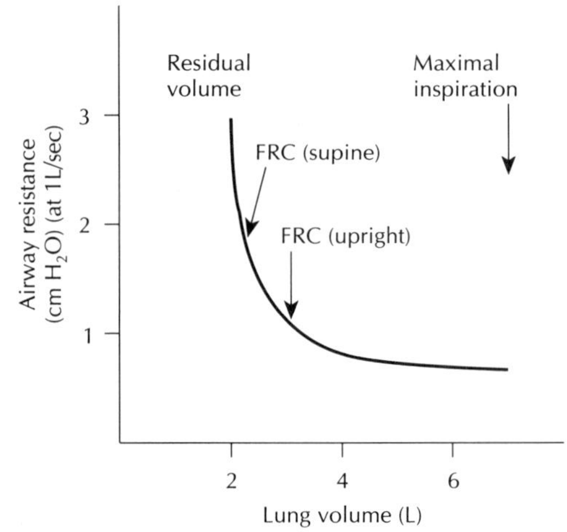


**FIG 40-1** Airway resistance is an increasingly hyperbolic function of decreasing lung volume. Functional residual capacity (FRC) decreases with changing from upright to supine position. (From Nunn JF. Applied Respiratory Physiology, 3rd ed. London: Butterworth-Heinemann Limited, 1987, p 64.)

vascular volume replacement was commenced with some improvement in blood pressure and heart rate. Repeat arterial blood gases revealed the following values: pH, 7.34; $Paco_2$, 58; $Pao_2$, 86. Ventilator settings were changed again as follows: tidal volume, 1000; respiratory rate, 6; $Fio_2$, 0.7. On these settings $P_{max}$ dropped to 32 cm $H_2O$, $P_{ei}$ was 20 cm $H_2O$, and intrinsic PEEP was 0. Expiratory rhonchi ceased prior to each breath. In spite of volume resuscitation, the PAOP had dropped to 8. A further dose of bronchodilators was administered. $P_{max}$ subsequently dropped to 28 cm $H_2O$; $P_{ei}$ remained at 20 cm $H_2O$. Arterial blood gases were: pH, 7.37; $Pco_2$, 52; $Po_2$, 105; and $Petco_2$ was 45. Multisystem resuscitation continued in the face of pulmonary sepsis and moderate hypotension.

Gas trapping is an extremely common problem in patients with obstructive lung disease. The consequent increased intrathoracic pressure often causes reduced venous return and subsequent hypotension. Although muscle paralysis is not universally necessary under these circumstances, in this case it was beneficial. It permitted early diagnosis of gas trapping by allowing machine airway pressure measurements to represent accurately patient status and by eliminating the confounding variable of diaphramatic contractions on intrathoracic pressure. While an esophogeal balloon or other method of measuring pleural pressure might have been useful in making a diagnosis without paralysis, accurate placement of such a monitor would have been very difficult under the circumstances. Two points deserve emphasis. First, gas trapping caused an increase in intrathoracic pressure, which, in addition to decreasing venous return, falsely elevated PAOP. To measure true transmural PAOP, one would have needed to measure pleural pressure. Second, $P_{max}$-$P_{ei}$ was 10 mm $H_2O$, well above the accepted value for normal and confirms increased resistance to flow. $P_{ei}$ dropped further than $P_{max}$ as gas trapping diminished, which is appropriate given the relationship between lung volume and airway resistance (Fig. 40-1). Note also that bronchodilators were effective in lowering $\Delta P$, a finding that suggests active bronchodilation and a lowering of resistance.

Increasing the tidal volume while lowering the respiratory rate accomplishes two things. First, it increases expiratory time, which allows better emptying of the lung. Second, the larger tidal volume may improve aveolar ventilation by providing sufficient volume to ventilate both highly compliant bullae and less compliant functioning lung.

# PART SEVEN

# *THE ART OF PRACTICE*

CHAPTER 41

# *Other Aspects of Patient Care*

Frank B. Cerra

## CASE 1

The patient was a 36-year-old woman with type I diabetes mellitus and many complications, including advancing peripheral neuropathy, advancing retinopathy with a declaration of being legally blind, and renal failure. After a short period of hemodialysis, she underwent successful renal transplantation and did well for several years. Peripheral arterial disease developed and progressed in her lower extremities, eventually necessitating bilateral above-knee amputations. On two previous occasions, 1 and 3 years prior to this admission, the patient had entered the SICU with an infection and had developed severe adult respiratory distress syndrome (ARDS) requiring 3 to 4 months of mechanical ventilation. In the year prior to this admission, her activity level had become severely restricted as a result of advancing neuropathy, retinopathy, and bilateral hand pain from arterial insufficiency that was not remediable with surgical therapy.

On this admission, the patient presented with another infection and again developed ARDS requiring mechanical ventilation. Her clinical course was one of multiple organ dysfunction. After 4 weeks her condition had stabilized, with normal liver function, renal insufficiency, and a stable ventilator status. Over the next 2 months, her pulmonary status did not improve. She was ventilator-dependent, required a large minute ventilation, demonstrated poor pulmonary compliance, and maintained reasonable arterial blood gases. On evaluation by her attending physician, consulting psychiatrist, health care personnel, and her mother, the patient's only relative, she was thought to be competent to make decisions.

The patient communicated through letter-pointing that she wanted all care withdrawn, including the ventilator, and that she wanted to be kept pain-free and allowed to die. A care conference was held with the patient, her mother, the medical and health care staff involved, the hospital chaplain, and the social worker who knew her well. The decision was made to continue support for 4 more weeks and then reevaluate. Appropriate chart notes were entered.

After 4 weeks, no substantial improvement in her status had occurred. The ventilation she required precluded her transfer to a chronic ventilator facility or to home. Another care conference was held and the decision was made to forego life-sustaining treatment.

After a meeting with the hospital chaplain, and with her mother present, analgesics and sedatives were administered to relieve pain and suffering. The ventilator was removed and the patient was extubated. Appropriate notations were made in the patient's chart by the attending physician. She expired peacefully.

This chapter can be studied in conjunction with *Essentials of Surgical Critical Care,* edited by Jerome H. Abrams and Frank B. Cerra (St. Louis: Quality Medical Publishing, Inc., 1993), Chapter 55.

## CASE 2

The patient was a 65-year-old woman with recurrent ovarian carcinoma in the abdomen, liver metastases, and lung metastases. She had entered the hospital for a course of chemotherapy. The patient had an advanced directive specifying that she did not want to be maintained on mechanical life support or to undergo CPR in the event of a cardiac or pulmonary arrest. Examination revealed massive ascites that was not responsive to fluid restriction or diuretic therapy and a left pleural effusion.

Approximately 4 days after her chemotherapy, she experienced the onset of progressive dyspnea. Diagnostic evaluation revealed a large pericardial effusion that was hemodynamically significant on ECHO. After talking with the patient and her husband, the decision was made to attempt a needle pericardiocentesis. During the procedure, gross blood was obtained, and the patient had cardiorespiratory arrest. Her husband wanted her treated, and she received CPR. She was immediately transported to the surgical suite, where an open drainage of the pericardium was performed. No bleeding site was found.

The patient was admitted to the SICU from the surgical suite. She was hemodynamically unstable. Fluids were administered, and a pulmonary artery catheter was placed. She was appropriately resuscitated and demonstrated adequate cardiac function. Over the next 2 to 3 days, she recovered and was discharged from the SICU. Five days later she was discharged from the hospital. She expired 6 months later at home.

# ABBREVIATIONS

| | | |
|---|---|---|
| Amyl | amylase | units/L |
| BP | blood pressure | mm Hg |
| BUN | blood urea nitrogen | mg/dl |
| Ca | calcium | mg/dl |
| CI | cardiac index | $L \cdot min^{-1} \cdot m^{-2}$ |
| Cl | chloride | mEq/L |
| CO | cardiac output | L/min |
| Cr | creatinine | mg/dl |
| CVP | central venous pressure | mm Hg |
| $Do_2$ | oxygen delivery | ml/min |
| $Dvo_2$ | arteriovenous oxygen content difference | vol% |
| Eos | eosinophil (count) | $10^3$ cells/$mm^3$ |
| $Fio_2$ | inspired fraction of oxygen | — |
| Glu | glucose | mg/dl |
| Hb | hemoglobin | g/dl |
| $HCO_3^-$ | bicarbonate | mEq/L |
| Hct | hematocrit | % |
| HR | heart rate, pulse | beats/min |
| I:E | ratio of inspiratory time to expiratory time | — |
| K | potassium | mEq/L |
| Lac | lactate | mmol |
| LDH | lactate dehydrogenase | units/L |
| MAP | mean airway pressure | cm/$H_2O$ |
| MAP | mean arterial pressure | mm Hg |
| Mg | magnesium | mEq/L |
| Na | sodium | mEq/L |
| P | pulse, heart rate | beats/min |
| PA | pulmonary artery pressure (systolic/diastolic) | mm Hg |
| Pa | arterial pressure (systolic/diastolic) | mm Hg |
| $Paco_2$ | arterial carbon dioxide partial pressure | mm Hg |
| $Pao_2$ | arterial oxygen partial pressure | mm Hg |
| PAP | peak airway pressure | cm $H_2O$ |
| PC-IRV | pressure-controlled inverse ratio ventilation | — |
| PCWP | pulmonary capillary wedge pressure | mm Hg |
| PEEP | positive end-expiratory pressure | cm $H_2O$ |
| $Petco_2$ | partial pressure of end-tidal carbon dioxide | mm Hg |
| plt | platelets | $10^5$ cells/$mm^3$ |
| $P_{pa}$ | pulmonary artery pressure (systolic/diastolic) | mm Hg |
| $P_{pao}$ | pulmonary artery occlusion pressure | mm Hg |

| | | |
|---|---|---|
| $P_{ra}$ | right atrial pressure | mm Hg |
| PVR | pulmonary vascular resistance | dyne · sec · $cm^{-5}$ |
| RA | right atrial pressure | mm Hg |
| RR | respiratory rate | breaths/min |
| RV | right ventricular pressure (systolic/diastolic) | mm Hg |
| $SaO_2$ | arterial oxygen saturation | % |
| SGOT | serum glutamic-oxaloacetic transaminase (aspartate aminotransferase) | units/L |
| $SpO_2$ | arterial oxygen saturation | % |
| SV | stroke volume | ml |
| SVR | systemic vascular resistance | dyne · sec · $cm^{-5}$ |
| SVRI | systemic vascular resistance index | dyne · sec · $cm^{-5}$ · $m^2$ |
| Trigly | triglycerides | mg/dl |
| TV | tidal volume | ml |
| UO | urine output | ml/hr |
| $VO_2$, $\dot{V}O_2$ | oxygen consumption index | ml/min/$m^2$ |
| $V_T$ | tidal volume | ml |
| WBC | white blood cell count | cells/$mm^3$ |